GENETICS – RESEARCH AND ISSUES

P53

STRUCTURE, FUNCTIONS AND ROLE IN DISEASE

GENETICS – RESEARCH AND ISSUES

Additional books and e-books in this series can be found
on Nova's website under the Series tab.

GENETICS – RESEARCH AND ISSUES

P53

STRUCTURE, FUNCTIONS AND ROLE IN DISEASE

MONTE STEVENS
EDITOR

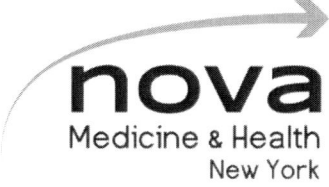

Copyright © 2020 by Nova Science Publishers, Inc.

All rights reserved. No part of this book may be reproduced, stored in a retrieval system or transmitted in any form or by any means: electronic, electrostatic, magnetic, tape, mechanical photocopying, recording or otherwise without the written permission of the Publisher.

We have partnered with Copyright Clearance Center to make it easy for you to obtain permissions to reuse content from this publication. Simply navigate to this **publication's** page on Nova's website and locate the "Get Permission" button below the title description. This button is linked directly to the title's permission page on copyright.com. Alternatively, you can visit copyright.com and search by title, ISBN, or ISSN.

For further questions about using the service on copyright.com, please contact:
Copyright Clearance Center
Phone: +1-(978) 750-8400   Fax: +1-(978) 750-4470   E-mail: info@copyright.com

NOTICE TO THE READER

The Publisher has taken reasonable care in the preparation of this book, but makes no expressed or implied warranty of any kind and assumes no responsibility for any errors or omissions. No liability is assumed for incidental or consequential damages in connection with or arising out of information contained in this book. The Publisher shall not be liable for any special, consequential, or exemplary damages resulting, in whole or in part, from the **readers'** use of, or reliance upon, this material. Any parts of this book based on government reports are so indicated and copyright is claimed for those parts to the extent applicable to compilations of such works.

Independent verification should be sought for any data, advice or recommendations contained in this book. In addition, no responsibility is assumed by the Publisher for any injury and/or damage to persons or property arising from any methods, products, instructions, ideas or otherwise contained in this publication.

This publication is designed to provide accurate and authoritative information with regard to the subject matter covered herein. It is sold with the clear understanding that the Publisher is not engaged in rendering legal or any other professional services. If legal or any other expert assistance is required, the services of a competent person should be sought. FROM A DECLARATION OF PARTICIPANTS JOINTLY ADOPTED BY A COMMITTEE OF THE AMERICAN BAR ASSOCIATION AND A COMMITTEE OF PUBLISHERS.

Additional color graphics may be available in the e-book version of this book.

Library of Congress Cataloging-in-Publication Data

ISBN: 978-1-53618-771-7

Published by Nova Science Publishers, Inc. † New York

CONTENTS

Preface		vii
Chapter 1	Function and Role of P53 in Hematologic Malignancies *Wei Cui*	1
Chapter 2	Mechanisms and Implication of p53 Mutation in Cancer *Eziafa I. Oduah and Steven R. Grossman*	83
Chapter 3	p53-Mediated Neuroprotective Effects of Natural Compounds in Oxidative Stress Conditions *Klara Zubčić, Goran Šimić and Maja Jazvinšćak Jembrek*	127
Index		183

PREFACE

p53: Structure, Functions and Role in Disease discusses the role of p53 dysregulation in different hematologic neoplasms defined by the current WHO classification. The prevalence of p53 aberration, mechanisms of p53 inactivation, regulation of p53 signaling pathway, and prognostic implications of p53 dysfunction in different hematologic malignancies are reviewed.

The authors also discuss the prevalence of p53 mutations in cancers and important mechanisms underlying the impact of p53 mutations such as loss of function, dominant negative effect and gain of function.

Recent findings related to the p53-mediated neuroprotective effects of natural compounds at the cellular, molecular, and behavioral level in various in vitro and in vivo models of neurodegenerative diseases are described, with a focus on Alzheimer's disease.

Chapter 1 - Dysfunctional p53 plays an important role in human tumorigenesis. *TP53* aberration occurs in 50-60% human solid tumors; however, the incidence of p53 aberration in hematologic malignancies can vary over a wide range, from 5% for low-grade B cell lymphomas such as extranodal marginal zone lymphoma of mucosa-associated lymphoid tissue or multiple myeloma (MM) at diagnosis to 50%-70% for MM at relapse or acute myeloid leukemia with complex karyotype. P53 aberration is associated with poor survival, disease progression, and low therapy response in hematologic malignancies. Multiple mechanisms of p53 dysregulation such as *TP53* deletion, *TP53* mutation, murine double minute 2/4 (MDM2/4) upregulation, ARF down-regulation, microRNA overexpression, epigenomic regulation, and post-translational modification are elucidated. In this review, the discussion is focused on the role of p53 dysregulation in different hematologic neoplasms defined by the current WHO classification. Prevalence of p53 aberration, mechanisms of p53 inactivation, regulation of p53 signaling pathway, and prognostic implication of p53 dysfunction in different hematologic malignancies will be discussed. Finally, current p53 targeted therapeutic approaches in different hematologic malignancies will be addressed.

Chapter 2 - Mutation of the *TP53* tumor suppressor gene, encoding the p53 protein, is found in nearly half of all human cancers, and is emerging as a potential therapeutic target. Missense mutant p53, in contrast to wildtype p53, can act as an oncogene, and is characterized by high stability and excess accumulation in cancer cells. Tumors harboring missense mutated p53 are dependent on its high level for its oncogenic functions that drive proliferation, invasion and metastasis. Therefore, the presence of oncogenic p53 mutations portends a poorer prognosis in certain cancers. In this chapter, the authors will discuss the prevalence of p53 mutation in cancers, as well as important mechanisms underlying the impact of p53 mutations, such as loss of function, dominant negative effect and gain of function. The authors also discuss the prognostic implications of mutant p53 in select cancer types and introduce emerging therapeutic approaches targeting this pathway in preclinical and clinical studies.

Chapter 3 - The transcription factor p53 orchestrates cellular response to different types of genotoxic challenges, including oxidative stress (OS). OS is induced by increased accumulation of reactive oxygen species and is tightly linked to the pathogenesis of various neurodegenerative diseases. During OS p53 undergoes posttranslational modifications that trigger its transcriptional activities, leading to activation of pro-apoptotic genes and repression of anti-apoptotic targets. In addition, p53 activity brings neurons into a more severe pro-oxidant condition based on the p53-driven activation of pro-oxidant genes and suppression of anti-oxidant genes. Recent studies suggest that dietary phytochemicals, such as flavonoids, may exert neuroprotective effects by downregulating expression of p53 gene *TP53* and acting along p53 pathways. In this chapter the authors will summarize recent findings related to the p53-mediated neuroprotective effects of natural compounds at the cellular, molecular, and behavioral level in various *in vitro* and *in vivo* models of neurodegenerative diseases, with a focus on Alzheimer's disease. Better understanding of the p53-mediated effects in neuroprotection may contribute to the development of more effective pharmacological approaches to OS-driven neurodegeneration.

In: p53
Editor: Monte Stevens

ISBN: 978-1-53618-771-7
© 2020 Nova Science Publishers, Inc.

Chapter 1

FUNCTION AND ROLE OF P53 IN HEMATOLOGIC MALIGNANCIES

*Wei Cui**
Department of Pathology and Laboratory Medicine,
University of Kansas Medical Center, Kansas City, KS 66160, US

ABSTRACT

Dysfunctional p53 plays an important role in human tumorigenesis. *TP53* aberration occurs in 50-60% human solid tumors; however, the incidence of p53 aberration in hematologic malignancies can vary over a wide range, from 5% for low-grade B cell lymphomas such as extranodal marginal zone lymphoma of mucosa-associated lymphoid tissue or multiple myeloma (MM) at diagnosis to 50%-70% for MM at relapse or acute myeloid leukemia with complex karyotype. P53 aberration is associated with poor survival, disease progression, and low therapy response in hematologic malignancies. Multiple mechanisms of p53 dysregulation such as *TP53* deletion, *TP53* mutation, murine double minute 2/4 (MDM2/4) upregulation, ARF down-regulation, microRNA overexpression, epigenomic regulation, and post-translational modification are elucidated. In this review, the discussion is focused on the role of p53 dysregulation in different hematologic neoplasms defined by

---

* Corresponding Author's E-mail: wcui@kumc.edu.

the current WHO classification. Prevalence of p53 aberration, mechanisms of p53 inactivation, regulation of p53 signaling pathway, and prognostic implication of p53 dysfunction in different hematologic malignancies will be discussed. Finally, current p53 targeted therapeutic approaches in different hematologic malignancies will be addressed.

Keywords: p53 aberration, MDM2, MDM4, ARF, p53 targeted therapy

INTRODUCTION

P53 is a tumor suppressor that maintains genomic integrity and stability through cell cycle arrest, DNA repair, and apoptosis (Levine 1997, Vousden and Lane 2007). Therefore, the p53 protein has been described as "the guardian of the genome". The *TP53* gene is located on chromosome 17p13 and defective *TP53* is one of the most common abnormalities detected in human cancers with a frequency of approximately 50% (Isobe et al. 1986, Levine and Oren 2009, Vogelstein and Kinzler 2004, Stengel et al. 2017). In hematologic neoplasms, the frequency of p53 alteration varies from 5% to 70%-80%. P53 dysregulation is related to disease progression, poor clinical outcomes, and insufficient therapeutic response in hematologic malignancies (Jovanovic et al. 2018, Kulasekararaj et al. 2013, Ok et al. 2015, Stengel et al. 2017, Wickremasinghe, Prentice, and Steele 2011).

Being at the helm of the cellular fate, both p53 expression and regulation are strictly controlled (Figure 1, regulation of p53). Under physiologic conditions, p53 is kept low through interaction with murine double minute 2 (MDM2). MDM2 regulates p53 stability via ubiquitination. MDM2 homo-oligomers have E3 ubiquitin ligase activity, which depends on an intact carboxy-terminal RING domain. When binding to p53, MDM2 ubiquitylates p53 and leads to its proteasomal degradation (Fang et al. 2000). p53 pathway is activated by cellular stress signals such as hypoxia, oxidative stress, nutritional deprivation, DNA damage, and oncogenic activation. Activation of p53 pathway is mediated by the protein stabilization, via the inhibition of a p53/murine MDM2 negative feedback loop or activation by p19ARF and cascade of ATM/CHK2/1 (Yu, Yu, and Young 2019, Kruse and Gu 2009).

The mechanisms by which ARF activates p53 function are complex (Chen, Yoon, and Gu 2010). ARF can stabilize nucleoplasmic p53 by binding MDM2 and sequestering it in the nucleolus (Weber et al. 1999). Nucleoplasmic forms of ARF can still activate p53 by directly inhibiting the ubiquitin ligase activity of MDM2 (Midgley et al. 2000, Llanos et al. 2001).

The activation of p53 pathway is further heightened through post-translational modifications including phosphorylation, acetylation, and methylation (Yue et al. 2017). Once activated, p53 binds to the p53 consensus DNA-binding elements usually located in the promoter and/or introns of its target genes and induces its downstream target genes (Figure 1, regulation of p53). These target genes are responsible for various functions including DNA damage response (*DNA damage protein-2 (DDB2)*, *XPC*), cell cycle arrest (*CDKN1A* and *GADD45*), apoptosis (*BAX*, *PUMA*, and *NOXA*), metabolism (*TP53- induced glycolysis and apoptosis regulator (TIGAR)* and *aldehyde dehydrogenase family 1 member A3*), and post-translational regulators of p53 (*MDM2* and *p53-induced phosphatase 1*) (Hafner et al. 2019). Interestingly, the interaction between p53 and MDM2 can be affected by stress status. In unstressed cells, ubiquitin specific protease 7 (USP7) deubiquitylates both p53 and MDM2 to keep a balanced state in which p53 is continuously degraded. However, under conditions of stress, the balance between p53 and its negative regulator is disrupted, resulting in p53 stabilization and apoptosis (Snaebjornsson and Schulze 2018). P53 pathway is also regulated by stress intensity. In response to weak or moderate stress insults, p53 stimulates expression of pro-survival genes that protect cells from damage in contrast to programmed cell death resulting from severe stress (Budanov 2014).

In addition to MDM2, murine double minute 4 (MDM4 or MDMX) has been identified as a protein sharing structural homology with MDM2 (Wade, Li, and Wahl 2013). By contrast, MDM4 does not homo-oligomerize and has no intrinsic ubiquitin ligase function but inactivates p53 by binding to and inhibiting the transactivation domain of p53 (Figure 1, regulation of p53). It can also increase MDM2 ubiquitin ligase activity as a stimulator (Linares et al. 2003). Hetero-oligomerization of MDM2 and MDM4 via their

RING domains may create a more effective p53 E3 ubiquitin ligase complex and is crucial for the suppression of p53 activity (Pant et al. 2011).

MicroRNAs (miRNAs) are small non-coding RNAs that regulate gene expression at the post-transcriptional level. Recent studies have demonstrated that miRNAs interact with p53 and its network at multiple levels. p53 regulates the transcription expression and the maturation of a group of miRNAs. p53 controls the expression of specific miRNAs to induce cell cycle arrest, senescence, and apoptosis, as well as to inhibit metastasis, angiogenesis, and glycolysis (Feng et al. 2011, Hermeking 2012, Liu et al. 2017). Mutant p53 upregulates expression of oncogenic miRNAs miR-128-2 through binding to the promoter of its host gene *ARPP21* in breast cancer cells to promote cell proliferation and cell survival (Li, Jones, et al. 2014). On the other hand, miRNAs regulate the activity and function of p53 through direct binding to 3' -UTR of the TP53 mRNA and downregulate its level and function (Hu et al. 2010, Feng et al. 2011, Suzuki et al. 2009, Liu et al. 2017). miR-125b and miR-504 are the first two miRNAs that were identified to directly target p53 (Le et al. 2009, Hu et al. 2010).

Recent studies have documented that some miRNAs indirectly regulate p53 through targeting regulators of p53 such as MDM2 and MDM4 (Liu et al. 2017, Hoffman, Pilpel, and Oren 2014). miR-192, miR-194, and miR-215 are found to directly target MDM2. Ectopic expression of these miRNAs in MM cell lines led to a reduction of MDM2 mRNA and protein and an increased level of p53 (Pichiorri et al. 2010). Another pair of MDM2-regulating miRNAs, miR-143 and miR-145, was found to be downregulated in head and neck squamous cell carcinoma compared to normal tissues and cells, while MDM2 was overexpressed in these tumors. *MDM2* is identified as a direct target of miR-143 and miR-145 (Zhang et al. 2013). miR-34a is also shown to target *MDM4*; specifically, miR-34a targets a conserved region of the MDM4 mRNA open reading frame (ORF) of exon 11, rather than its 3'UTR (Mandke et al. 2012). Another miRNA that targets *MDM4* directly is miR-10a, which was upregulated in *NPM1*-mutant AML. NPM1 stabilizes p53 in the nucleus when DNA damage occurs (Ovcharenko et al. 2011). miR-191-5p, miR-887, miR-661, miR-199a-3p, and let-7 repress *MDM4* through directly targeting the 3' -UTR of MDM4 (Liu et al. 2017).

STRUCTURE OF P53

p53 is a 393 amino acid/53 KD nuclear phosphoprotein composed of several functional domains (Levine 1997, (Hafner et al. 2019). p53 protein has five domains: two N-terminal transactivation domains that interact with transcriptional machinery to modulate the expression of growth regulatory genes; a proline-rich region which plays a role in DNA repair in response to γ-radiation and contribution to transcription activation; a sequence-specific DNA-binding domain that binds to the promoter area of target genes and hotpot for the most of tumor-derived missense mutations; an oligomerization domain that mediates the formation of homo- and hetero-tetramers of p53 protein; and finally a C-terminal region necessary for nuclear localization and non-specific DNA binding (Figure 2, structure of p53).

TP53 ABERRATIONS

TP53 abnormalities include mutation and deletion. *TP53* mutations in hematologic malignancies are detected in exons 5 to 8, which encode the DNA-binding domain of the protein, with a small number found in exon 4 (Cheung, Horsman, and Gascoyne 2009, Prokocimer et al. 1998). The most common alteration are missense mutations, followed by deletions and insertions, nonsense, silent, and splicing mutations (Prokocimer et al. 1998). In all types of human cancers, the missense *TP53* mutations are identified predominantly in 6 hotspot residues located within the DNA-binding domain (residues R175, G245, R248, R249, R273, and R282, Figure 2, structure of p53) (Herrero et al. 2016).

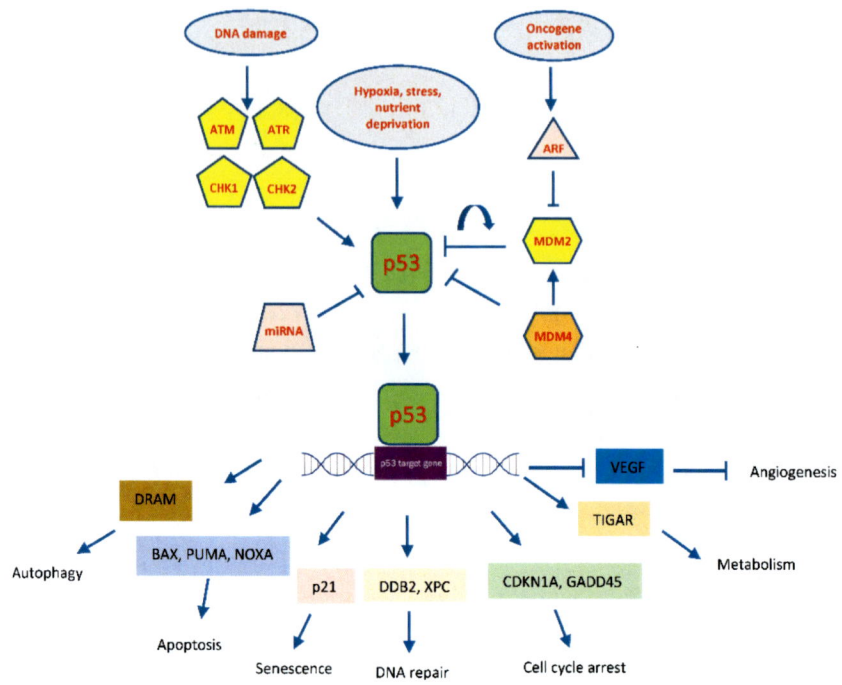

Figure 1. Regulation of p53. p53 is activated by DNA damage, oncogenic activation, hypoxia, stress, and nutritional deprivation. P53 signaling pathway is regulated by ARF, MDM2, MDM4, and miRNAs. Once p53 is activated, it binds to p53 target genes and stimulates their downstream events.

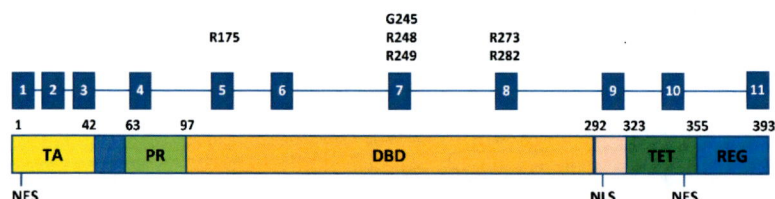

Figure 2. Structure of p53. *TP53* gene is composed of 11 exons. The hotspot mutations are located between exons 5-8. P53 protein is composed of N-terminal transactivation domains (TA), proline-rich domain (PD), a sequence-specific DNA-binding domain (DBD), an oligomerization domain (TET), and a C-terminal regulatory region (REG) with nuclear localization signal (NLS) and nuclear export signal (NES).

Deletion of the chromosomal region 17p13, containing the *TP53* gene locus is often associated with inferior prognosis, poor response to chemotherapy, and advanced stage in multiple myeloma (MM) and chronic lymphocytic leukemia/small lymphocytic lymphoma (CLL/SLL) patients. Both *TP53* mutations and deletions are found to associate with complex karyotypes (CK) in acute myeloid leukemia (AML), acute lymphoblastic leukemia/lymphoma (ALL) and myelodysplastic syndrome (MDS) (Stengel et al. 2017).

Li–Fraumeni syndrome (LFS) is a rare autosomal dominant cancer predisposition syndrome caused by germline *TP53* gene mutations (Bougeard et al. 2008). Patients with LFS show increased risk of developing solid tumors and hematologic malignancies including ALL and therapy-related MDS/ therapy-related AML (t-MDS/t-AML) (Swaminathan et al. 2019). Although most patients with hematologic malignancy and LFS can obtain an initial response to induction therapy, sustained responses are not able to be achieved, and outcomes are extremely poor. *TP53*-mutated lymphocytes in patients with LFS are demonstrated to show intrinsic resistance to conventional chemotherapeutic drugs (Swaminathan et al. 2019).

P53 IN MYELOID NEOPLASMS

TP53 in Clonal Hematopoiesis

Clonal hematopoiesis (CH) defines an age-associated progressive expansion of a clonal population of blood cells with one or more somatic mutations derived from a single hematopoietic stem cell (HSC) clone (Bowman, Busque, and Levine 2018). Although many somatic mutations may be selection neutral, HSCs will retain mutations that provide advantages for self-renewal, blocking differentiation, and resolving DNA damage without apoptosis induction. This growth benefit results in an expansion of the HSC clones that carry the favored somatic mutations (Barbosa et al. 2019). Individuals with CH have a higher risk for hematological malignancies and cardiovascular events (Bowman, Busque, and Levine 2018).

TP53 plays an important role in CH. *TP53* mutation is one of the most common mutations in CH, in addition to mutations in *DNMT3A*, *TET2*, *ASXL1*, *JAK2*, *PPM1D*, *SF3B1*, *SRSF2*, *CBL*, and *GNB1* (Bowman, Busque, and Levine 2018, Desai et al. 2018, Gibson and Steensma 2018). These mutations are initiating events that cause clonal hematopoietic expansion (Xie, Lu, et al. 2014). Selective pressure such as aging or chemoradiation therapy can drive the emergence of HSC clones enriched with *TP53* mutation, which offers a fitness advantage in the face of genotoxic stress.

Aging is associated with a number of hematological complications including anemia, defective innate and adaptive immunity, and increased risk in developing myeloid neoplasms (Bowman, Busque, and Levine 2018). A recent study has showed that *TP53* mutant clones are enriched in anemia cohort. These findings suggest *TP53* clones in the context of anemia may have gained survival benefit in response to extrinsic environmental stressors, such as inflammation (van Zeventer et al. 2020). Wong et al. found that *TP53* mutations were present at a higher incidence in t-AML patients than in de novo AML patients (Wong et al. 2015). Importantly, the number of total mutations did not significantly differ between these two groups, indicating a lack of mutagenic activity induced by chemotherapy. Instead, in several patients, *TP53* mutations were found to be present in the blood prior to the onset of disease. These findings provide clear evidence that *TP53* mutations may offer a survival advantage upon genotoxic stress and lead to clonal expansion in t-AML. Another recent study in animal models also demonstrates that mutant p53 confers a competitive advantage to HSC clone for its expansion after radiation-induced stress (Chen et al. 2019).

Desai P et al. conducted mutational profiling on 212 blood samples taken years before the diagnosis of AML (Desai et al. 2018). In their findings, *TP53*, *IDH1*, *IDH2* or *RUNX1* with *PHF6* mutations exhibited increased specificity and penetrance for the development of AML. A rapid rise in the allelic fraction of *IDH2* or *TP53* mutations was significantly associated with a shorter time in progress to AML. Their study also revealed the stepwise acquisition of mutations leading to AML. *TP53*, *NPM1*, and

SRSF2 mutants emerged in dominant subclones preceding the development of AML, whereas CH associated *DNMT3A* and *TET2* mutants were maintained over time. This study further emphasizes the importance of *TP53* mutations associated with CH in AML development.

TP53 Aberration in Acute Myeloid Leukemia

AML is a genetically heterogeneous clonal HSC malignancy characterized by chromosomal abnormalities, genetic mutations, epigenetic modifications, and miRNA deregulations. Despite progress in understanding AML pathogenesis and emerging novel therapies, AML continues to be an aggressive malignancy with high morbidity and mortality (Prokocimer, Molchadsky, and Rotter 2017). The frequency of *TP53* mutation in de novo AML is 4.5%-15% (Peller and Rotter 2003, Zhang et al. 2017), but can be as high as 27%-40% in t-AML and 50-70% AML with complex karyotype (CK) (Peller and Rotter 2003, Zhang et al. 2017, Daneshbod et al. 2019).

The most common mutations are missense mutations occurring in the DNA binding-domain (encoded by exons 5–8) with a predilection for arginine residues and noted mutational "hot-spots" such as R175H, Y220C, R248Q, and R273C (Hunter and Sallman 2019). The frameshift mutations, in-frame, splice-site, and nonsense mutations are less frequent (Stengel et al. 2017). While two-thirds of missense mutations of *TP53* frequently yield loss-of-function (LOF) phenotypes and exert dominant-negative effects over the remaining wild-type allele (Brosh and Rotter 2009), some mutant alleles can modulate gene transcription defined as "gain-of-function" (GOF) (Milner, Medcalf, and Cook 1991, Prokocimer, Molchadsky, and Rotter 2017). Somatic *TP53* LOF mutations promote HSC cell clonal expansion and drive AML initiation (Prokocimer, Molchadsky, and Rotter 2017). GOF mutants promote chemoresistance, invasiveness, and tumor cell proliferation. Another function of GOF demonstrated in *TP53*^{R175H} is its ability to promote aberrant self-renewal in leukemic cells, a function that is present in hematopoietic stem and progenitor cells (Loizou et al. 2019). *TP53* mutations are highly associated with older age, 17p abnormality, complex cytogenetics, and monosomy 5 and 7 in AML patients (Zhang et al. 2017). *TP53* mutations appear to be mutually exclusive of other mutations including *NPM1*, *FLT3-ITD*, and *DNMT3A* (Daneshbod et al. 2019).

Overall survival (OS) is significantly poorer in AML patients with *TP53* aberrations (Stengel et al. 2017). A high mutation burden with a variant allele of fraction (VAF) of >50% confers a negative impact on OS. Grossmann and colleagues demonstrated that *TP53* mutation was an independent prognostic factor for both OS and event-free survival (EFS) in AML patients (Grossmann et al. 2012). Even in the CK cohort, those with *TP53* mutations had an inferior outcome, with a 3-year OS of 0% vs. 27.9% (Grossmann et al. 2012). Likewise, AML patients with 17p abnormality show a 3-year OS of 15% and a cumulative incidence of relapse of 49% at 3 years (Middeke et al. 2014). Furthermore, almost 70% of all relapses occur within the first 6 months after allogeneic stem cell transplant.

P53 Protein Overexpression in AML

p53 expression is used as a surrogate marker of *TP53* mutation in MDS and AML (Cleven et al. 2015, Saft et al. 2014, McGraw et al. 2016). Similar to *TP53* mutation, p53 expression is shown to significantly associate with MDS patients with high-risk cytogenetic abnormalities and AML patients with myelodysplastic related changes, carrying complex karyotypes, and *TP53* mutations (Cleven et al. 2015, McGraw et al. 2016). p53 expression confers a negative impact on OS in patients with therapy-related myeloid neoplasms and MDS and relapse-free survival (RFS) in patients with de novo AML (Cleven et al. 2015, Saft et al. 2014, Molteni et al. 2019, Assi et al. 2018, Pich, Godio, and Davico Bonino 2017, Fernandez-Pol et al. 2017). Our recent study confirms the same findings in AML and MDS patients (Gao et al. 2020).

P53 Pathway Dysregulation in AML

p53 inactivation more often results from the overexpression of its endogenous inhibitors MDM2 or MDM4, which frequently occurs in p53 wild-type (WT) AML (Quesnel et al. 1994, Seliger et al. 1996). Early studies reported that MDM2 mRNA and protein overexpression were present in about half of AML cases (Bueso-Ramos et al. 1993, Bueso-Ramos et al. 1995, Seliger et al. 1996), whereas *MDM2* amplification was not detected in any of these cases (Bueso-Ramos et al. 1993, Quesnel et al. 1994). p53 mRNA overexpression is also correlated with MDM2 mRNA overexpression (Seliger et al. 1996). MDM2 overexpressed AML patients have shorter EFS and a trend for shorter clinical remission (CR) (Faderl et al. 2000). A recent study has documented that MDM4 mRNA and protein overexpression are present in 100% and 92% of AML cases, respectively (Han et al. 2016). AML patients with CK and WT *TP53* are found to have increased MDM4 mRNA expression compared to normal karyotype (NK) AML patients. Karyotype analysis in MDM4 overexpressed cell lines detects aneuploidy and polyploidy that result from MDM4 overexpression. These findings suggest the important role of MDM4 overexpression plays in pathogenesis of CK-AML with WT *TP53* by inhibiting p53-signal pathway (Li et al. 2014).

ARF, encoded in the *Cdkn2a* locus, a major WT p53 positive regulator, antagonizes its MDM2-dependent degradation. *ARF* deletion is uncommon in AML (5%), which is associated with poorer clinical outcomes (Faderl et al. 2000). Low ARF expression is more frequent (>40%), due to suppression by AML1-ETO fusion protein in AML with t(8;21) or increased degradation secondary to mutant nucleophosmin (NPM) in AML with *NPM1* mutation (Linggi et al. 2002, Colombo et al. 2006, Prokocimer, Molchadsky, and Rotter 2017). Low ARF level predicts poorer OS in AML patients (Muller-Tidow et al. 2004). Transcriptional repression of ARF is also modulated by DNA methylation of *Cdkn2a* in AML (Paul et al. 2010). Homeobox gene *Hhex* regulates the development of HSCs (Argiropoulos and Humphries 2007). High HHEX expression has been reported in AML patients, regardless of leukemia subtype, with highest expression found in AML with inv(16)/t(16;16) or t(8;21) translocations (Shields et al. 2016). HHEX directly binds to *Cdkn2a* locus and enables H3K27mes-mediated epigenetic repression of *Cdkn2a*. Conditional deletion of *Hhex* leads to up-regulation of p16INK4a and p19ARF in cell lines (Shields et al. 2016).

miRNA and p53 Interaction in AML

miRNAs and p53 interact with each other. miRNAs function as regulators as well as targets of p53. miR-125b, a negative regulator of p53 (Le et al. 2009), was one of the most overexpressed miRNAs of the 32 differentially expressed miRNAs examined in a study of cytogenetically-normal (CN) AML patients 60-year or older (Whitman et al. 2010). miR-3151 is another negative regulator of p53 (Lankenau et al. 2015). High miR-3151 expression was identified in a study of 179 CN-AML patients, which was associated with shorter disease-free survival and OS (Eisfeld et al. 2012). Subsequently, overexpression of miR-3151 was found to reduce the abundance of *TP53* mRNA and p53 protein by directly targeting the 3′UTR of *TP53*, which resulted in reduced apoptosis and chemoresistance in AML cell lines (Eisfeld et al. 2014). As miR-34a is a direct target of p53, miR-34a expression is reduced in AML cases with CK and biallelic *TP53* alterations. Low expression of miR-34a is associated with inferior OS, RFS, and chemoresistance (Rucker et al. 2013).

TP53 Aberration in Myelodysplastic Syndrome

MDS is a heterogenous group of HSC malignancies characterized by cytopenia, ineffective hematopoiesis, and risk of AML transformation. The incidence of *TP53* mutation in MDS is low, in the range of 5-9% (Kulasekararaj et al. 2013, Stengel et al. 2017). *TP53* mutations are reported to be exclusively associated with isolated 5q- and CK with -5/5q- in MDS patients (Kulasekararaj et al. 2013). The prevalence of *TP53* mutations is also higher in t-MDS and t-AML compared to de novo MDS and AML (37%

vs. 14.5%) (Ok et al. 2015). 17p deletion is enriched in MDS patients with CK (65%, 15/23 cases), but not identified in any MDS cases with isolated del(5q) or one additional abnormality (Sebaa et al. 2012). The incidence of abnormalities of chromosome 17 was 11.9% in a study of 271 MDS patients (Marisavljevic et al. 2004), while it was reduced to 2.0% in a large cohort study of 2,072 MDS patients. -17/17p- was again enriched in cases with CK (95.2%) in the latter study (Haase 2008).

5q deletion in MDS leads to dysregulation of p53 pathway. Deletion of the long arm of chromosome 5 causes the loss of 1.5 megabases of the "commonly deleted region" (CDR), which is composed of 41 genes situated at or near 5q32-33 (Zhang et al. 2017, Cumbo et al. 2020, Lee, List, and Sallman 2019). These important genes include *RSP14*, *miR145* and *miR146*, *CDC25c/PP2A*, *SPARC*, *HSPA9*, *CD74*, *EGR1*, and *DIAPH*. Using an RNA interference approach to target and silence each gene of CDR, Ebert et al. found that only *RPS14* suppression recapitulated the del(5q) phenotype *in vitro* (Ebert et al. 2008, Ebert 2009). *RPS14* suppression by shRNAs resulted in p53 accumulation in primary human hematopoietic progenitor cells and cell lines (Dutt et al. 2011). Nucleolar stress arising from *RPS14* deficiency increased the levels of free, unbound, small ribosomal proteins, RPL11. Subsequently, RPL11 bound MDM2 and interfered MDM2-p53 interaction, which led to p53 activation (Dutt et al. 2011). Conditional inactivation of *Rps14* in mice resulted in an erythroid differentiation defect mediated by p53 activation that was induced by proteins involved in innate immunity signaling (Schneider et al. 2016).

TP53 aberrations carry significant prognostic impact. *TP53* mutation is positively correlated with p53 expression, high blast count, leukemic progression, and refractoriness to Lenalidomide treatment (Jadersten et al. 2011, Haase et al. 2019, Kulasekararaj et al. 2013). Patients with *TP53* mutations had shorter median OS compared to patients with WT *TP53* (9 months vs. 66 months) (Kulasekararaj et al. 2013). Furthermore, the presence of *TP53* mutation in MDS patients with CK further divided this group of patients into distinct prognostic subgroups (Haase et al. 2019). *TP53*-mutated group was associated with monosomal karyotype, high CK defined by carrying five or more karyotypic abnormalities, fewer somatic mutations, and shorter median OS of 0.6 years. MDS patients with *TP53* mutation had short response duration to hypomethylating agents (HMAs) compared to patients with WT *TP53* (Takahashi et al. 2016).

TP53 mutation burden also influences survival and treatment response to HMAs in MDS (Montalban-Bravo et al. 2020, Sallman et al. 2016). A *TP53* VAF >40% was a prognostic indicator for poorer OS in univariant and multivariant analyses (Sallman et al. 2016). Lower *TP53* mutation VAF correlated with higher overall response rate (ORR), but there were no differences in CR rate or response duration based on VAF. i(17p) or 17p-MDS belongs to the intermediate risk group (Sole et al. 2005, Greenberg et al. 2012). *TP53* deletion is associated with poorer OS compared to WT *TP53* (24 months vs. 65 months) (Stengel et al. 2017) and lower ORR to HMAs (Montalban-Bravo et al. 2020).

As we discussed in previous AML section, p53 overexpression is documented to have a positive association with *TP53* mutation (McGraw et al. 2016, Kulasekararaj et al. 2013, Jadersten et al. 2011) and predicts poor clinical outcomes (Saft et al. 2014, McGraw et al. 2016, Molteni et al. 2019). Saft el al. found that strong p53 expression in ≥ 1% of bone marrow cells was significantly associated with higher risk of leukemic transformation (P = 0.0006), shorter OS (P = 0.0175), and a lower cytogenetic response rate (P = 0.009), but not with achievement or duration of 26-week transfusion independence response and served as an independent predictor for leukemic progression (Saft et al. 2014). Another study also showed that p53 expression was positively correlated with chromosome17 abnormalities, high blast count, high *TP53* mutation burden, and inferior OS (McGraw et al. 2016). Due to its prognostic implication, a Japanese group proposed a new prognostic index that applied combined p53 expression and cytogenetics to evaluation of short-term prognosis in MDS patients treated with azacytidine (Nishiwaki et al. 2016). p53 expression is also found to be associated with MDS with marrow fibrosis regardless of mutational status and shorter OS (Loghavi et al. 2015, Ramos et al. 2016). These collective findings support that p53 immunohistochemical study may be considered as a reliable screening tool for the detection of *TP53* mutations in MDS or a reasonable alternative when the *TP53* sequencing technologies are not available (McGraw et al. 2016, Cumbo et al. 2020).

TP53 Mutation in Myeloproliferative Neoplasms

Myeloproliferative neoplasms (MPN) are chronic hematopoietic disorders characterized by clonal proliferation of mature myeloid elements. In chronic phase of MPN, the frequency of p53 defects is low; in contrast, they are more frequent in post-MPN AML. The prevalence of *TP53* mutation is reported to be as low as 4% in primary myelofibrosis, but goes up to 11% in blast phase of MPN (Tefferi and Pardanani 2015). *JAK2V617F* mutation often co-occurs with *TP53* mutation in leukemic transformed MPN. The VAF of *TP53* is also significantly higher in post-MPN AML samples than in MPN samples (7% versus 57%, respectively, $P < 0.01$). The VAF of *TP53* mutation markedly increases at the time of leukemic transformation, whereas the VAF of concurrent *ASXL1* and *IDH2* mutations does not increase (Rampal et al. 2014). *TP53* mutation expansion during MPN transformation into AML is a multistep process. NGS analyses on serial samples of MPN patients found that low allelic burden of *TP53* mutations was present for a few years in the chronic MPN phase, whereas after loss of the WT *TP53* allele, the p53 mutant clone rapidly increased, resulting in leukemic progression (Lundberg et al. 2014).

Chemotherapy in p53 Mutated AML and MDS

Standard 7+3 induction therapy is associated with dismal clinical outcomes with increased recurrent rate and poor OS in p53 mutated AML patients (Hunter and Sallman 2019). Recent works show that the HMAs azacitidine and decitabine are the preferred frontline treatment compared to standard therapy. In the AZA-AML-001 study (NCT01074047) (Dohner et al. 2018), *TP53* mutations only demonstrated a negative impact on OS in the conventional care treatment group while *TP53* mutated patients treated with azacitidine showed an improved median OS of 7.2 months compared to 2.4 months in the standard care group (p = 0.09). The same study also found that azacytidine treated AML patients with abnormal 17p showed a trend of superior OS (p = 0.07) compared to patients treated with conventional therapy. Welch et al. exhibited that decitabine treated AML and MDS patients with *TP53* mutations had a marked response rate with robust mutation and blast clearance (defined by VAF and blast count < 5%, respectively) (NCT01687400) (Welch et al. 2016).

Rescuing Wild-Type p53 Inactivation

The frequency of *TP53* mutations remains low in de novo and/or non-CK AML. However, functional inactivation of p53 or of its pathway appears to be a requisite for transformation. Recent study indicates most AML may bear other aberrations that can deleteriously influence the function and activity of WT p53, including MDM2/MDM4 upregulation, ARF downregulation, deregulated post-translational modification, up/down-stream signaling aberration, and miRNA deregulation (Prokocimer, Molchadsky, and Rotter 2017).

The reactivation of intact p53 activity which results in restoration of intrinsic apoptotic pathway has risen as an encouraging therapeutic strategy (Cassier et al. 2017, Barbosa et al. 2019). There are several approaches to take in term of reactivation of p53 pathway (Andreeff et al. 2016). MDM2 overexpression has been reported in up to 50% of AML (Quintás-Cardama et al. 2017). One such scheme is to utilize MDM2/4 inhibitors that directly block the MDM2-p53 interaction (Figure 3A, p53 targeted therapy). The breakthrough came in 2004 with the discovery of the Nutlins by Vassilev et al. (Vassilev et al. 2004) which opened the gateway for efficiently targeting this pathway in the clinic. Several classes of small molecules that selectively bind to MDM2 by mimicking these amino acids and activate WT p53 in a nongenotoxic manner have been investigated (Moll and Petrenko 2003, Cassier et al. 2017, Vassilev et al. 2004, Herrero et al. 2016, Richmond J 2015, Salmoiraghi, Rambaldi, and Spinelli 2018). These studies have led to several clinical trials with RG7112, RG-7388/Idasanutlin, AMG-232, DS-3032b/Milademetan, and HDM201 (Erba et al. 2019, Andreeff et al. 2016, Khurana and Shafer 2019, Ravandi et al. 2016).

The first MDM2 inhibitor to progress into human clinical trials is RG7112 (Hoffmann La Roche RO5045337) (Vu et al. 2013). In a phase 1 trial (NCT00623870), RG7112 was administered to 116 patients including relapsed/refractory AML (R/R AML), CR and partial response (PR) were observed in 3 and 2 out of 30 evaluable AML patients (Andreeff et al. 2016).

RG7388 (Idasanutlin) is a second-generation MDM2 inhibitor and is more potent and selective than RG7112 (Ding et al. 2013). In a multicenter phase 1/1b study, RG7388 (idasanutlin) was evaluated in 86 AML patients as monotherapy and in combination with cytarabine. CRs occurred rapidly and were durable (> 60 d) in elderly AML patients with RG7388 monotherapy and in R/R AML patients with combination therapy (Yee K. et al. 2014). This study has advanced to phase 3 clinical trial (NCT02545283).

AMG 232, a potent oral MDM2 inhibitor, has also been evaluated in adults with R/R AML. In a phase 1b trial, AMG 232 with or without trametinib (MEK inhibitor) was administered to 36 R/R AML patients (NCT02016729). Of 30 evaluable patients, 1 achieved CR, 4 achieved morphologic leukemia-free state, and 1 achieved PR (Erba et al. 2019).

DS-3032b (milademetan) is an oral p53-MDM2 inhibitor currently under evaluation in patients with AML and other hematological malignancies. In phase 1 dose-escalation study in 38 patients with R/R AML and high-risk MDS (NCT02319369), CR was achieved in 2 AML patients, with a remission duration of >4 and >10 months, respectively. One MDS patient achieved marrow CR with platelet improvement, with 4 months duration (DiNardo et al. 2016).

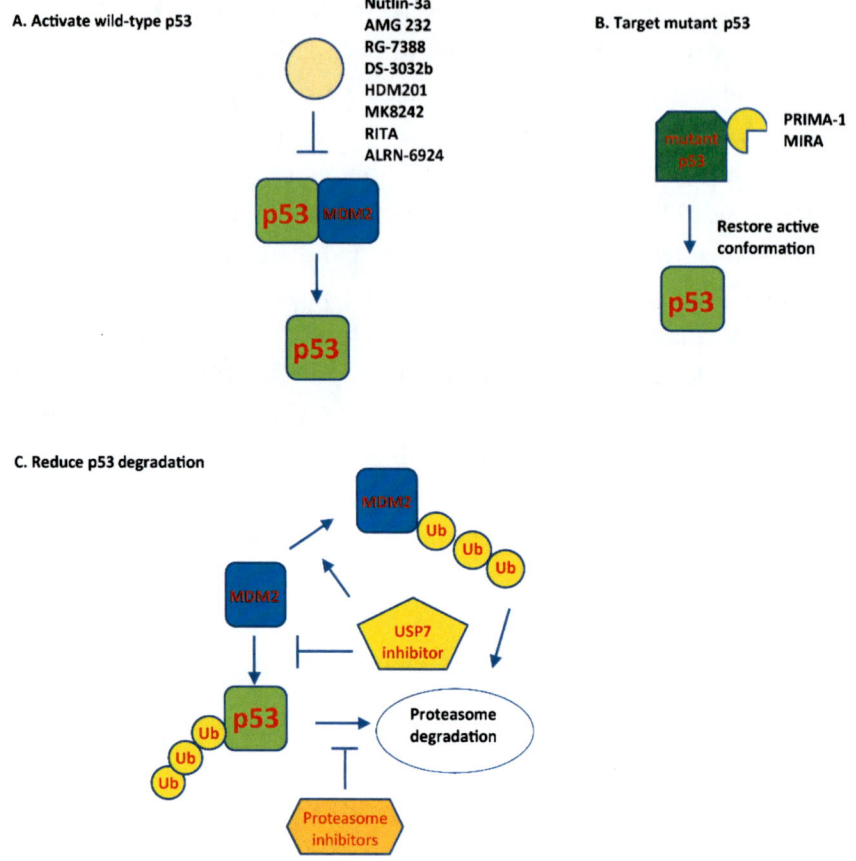

Figure 3. p53 targeted therapy. A. MDM2 inhibitors disrupt MDM2-p53 interaction and activate wild-type p53. B. PRIMA-1 and MIRA restore active conformation of mutant p53. C. Proteasome inhibitors block p53 degradation in proteasome and enhance p53 activity. USP7 inhibitor promotes MDM2 degradation and increases p53 activity.

HDM201, an oral MDM2 inhibitor as monotherapy has been evaluated in 37 R/R AML and 2 R/R ALL patients in a multicentric phase 1 clinical trial (NCT02143635). An ORR was 20.6% including 3 CR and 4 CR with Incomplete Hematologic Recovery (CRi) (Stein et al. 2017).

MK8242 is a potent, orally bioavailable, small-molecule MDM2 inhibitor. A phase 1 clinical trial on 26 R/R AML patients showed a more favorable safety profile but a limited clinical response (Ravandi et al. 2016)

(NCT01451437). This clinical trial was terminated early due to business reasons.

A recent study shows MDM4 mRNA and protein overexpression are present in 100% and 92% of AML cases, respectively (Han et al. 2016). MDM4 mRNA is also found to be overexpressed in HSC and granulocyte-monocytic progenitor-enriched (GMP) cells from AML patients compared to healthy control patients (Carvajal et al. 2018). Due to these indispensable and nonoverlapping roles in suppressing the normal function of p53 played by MDM2 and MDM4, dual inhibition of MDM2 and MDM4 might be required for full TP53 activation. These findings lead to the investigation of potential therapeutic effect of a stapled alpha-helical cell-penetrating peptide, ALRN-6924, a dual inhibitor of MDM2 and MDM4, in AML. This peptide is shown to robustly activate p53 pathway, inhibit AML cell growth via induction of cell cycle arrest and apoptosis, and exert robust antileukemic effects *in vitro* and *in vivo* (Carvajal et al. 2018). An ongoing phase 1/1b study of the ALRN-6924, a dual inhibitor of MDM4 and MDM2, as monotherapy or in combination with cytarabine for the treatment of relapsed/refractory AML and advanced MDS with WT *TP53*, showed clinical activity and an acceptable safety profile (Sallman, Borate, et al. 2018).

Targeting Mutant p53

Directly or indirectly targeting mutant p53 is an innovative tactic that is particularly effective due to its specificity against the underlying biology of the disease (Figure 3B, p53 targeted therapy). APR-246/PRIMA-1^{MET} (APR-246), a methylated derivative of PRIMA-1, functions to restore active conformation and activity of mutant p53. APR-246 induced apoptosis in *TP53* mutant AML cells resulting from caspase activation and cell cycle arrest (Nahi et al. 2006). APR-246 synergized with azacitidine to induce cell cycle arrest and apoptosis in AML/MDS cell lines and primary cells from MDS and AML patients (Maslah et al. 2019). The first-in-human study with this compound reduced blast count from 46% to 26% in the bone marrow of the one AML patient on the study carrying a *TP53* core domain mutation (Lehmann et al. 2012).

Preliminary results of a phase 1b/2 trial of combined APR-246 and azacitidine in MDS and AML patients demonstrated tolerability of this regimen and promising clinical response with a CR rate of 82% and deep molecular remissions (Sallman, DeZern, et al. 2018). The same phase 2 clinical trial in a very high-risk elderly populations of French patients found that combined therapy demonstrated a promising 56% CR rate at 6 cycles and a deep molecular remission in all CR patients (Cluzeau et al. 2019). This phase 2 trial in American patients with *TP53* mutant MDS and oligoblastic AML showed an ORR of 87% and CR rate of 61% and 50% for MDS and AML, respectively. A high fraction of cytogenetic and deep molecular remissions was also achieved, which led to subsequent stem cell transplant and an improved OS (Sallman et al. 2019). This trial is ongoing and a multi-center, randomized phase 3 trial has recently opened for recruitment (NCT03745716).

TP53 ABERRATIONS IN ACUTE LYMPHOBLASTIC LEUKEMIA/LYMPHOMA

Acute lymphoblastic leukemia/lymphoma (ALL) is an aggressive clonal disease of B- or T-cell origin characterized by biologic and clinical heterogeneity and affects both children and adults. *TP53* mutations have been investigated in both pediatric and adult ALL patients. The studies conducted in children affected by ALL conclude that *TP53* alterations including mutation and deletion are present at a much higher frequency at relapse, accounting for 12.5% in B-ALL and 6.4% in T-ALL if compared to the incidence at diagnosis (Hof et al. 2011, Salmoiraghi, Rambaldi, and Spinelli 2018). More than half of the mutations emerge at relapse. *TP53* alteration predicts poor EFS, poor OS and poor response to chemotherapy in pediatric ALL cases (Hof et al. 2011, Krentz et al. 2013). A recent study performed on 111 Taiwan pediatric ALL patients confirmed higher incidence of *TP53* alterations in 29% and 46% B- and T-ALL cases at relapse and more than 70% of *TP53* aberrations gained at the relapse (Yu et al. 2020). The incidence was much elevated than similar studies in Caucasian children. *TP53* alterations were again associated with poor 5-year EFS and 5-year OS.

In contrast to relatively low frequency of *TP53* mutations at 2-3% in pediatric ALL at diagnosis (Wada et al. 1993, Kawamura et al. 1999), adult ALL patients demonstrate higher incidence of *TP53* mutations. A study on 98 adult ALL patients showed *TP53* mutations detected in 8.2% of these patients, representing 6.4% and 11.1% B- and T-ALL, respectively (Chiaretti et al. 2013). The largest series study of 625 newly diagnosed pediatric and adult ALL patients revealed a higher incidence of *TP53* mutations of 15.7% of entire cohort, partially due to inclusion of Burkitt lymphoma (BL) (Stengel et al. 2014). *TP53* mutations occurred in 15.4% B-ALL and less frequently in 7.6% T-ALL. The vast majority of mutations were missense mutations (81.8%), followed by frameshift (7.2%), in-frame (4.5%), splice-site (2.7%), and nonsense mutations (3.6%) and affected preferentially in DNA-binding domain and known hotspots (Stengel et al. 2014).

TP53 mutations positively associate with hypodiploidy and *MLL* rearranged ALL, older patients and negatively associate with ALL with *BCR-ABL1* translocation. *TP53* mutations are also frequently correlated with *TP53* deletion on the second allele, further confirming the "second hit" theory of tumor suppressor genes and their roles in cancer pathogenesis. The analysis on the clinical impact of the *TP53* alteration performed by Stengel A et al. revealed that the OS was dramatically worse in patients with *TP53* mutation, deletion or combined abnormalities (Stengel et al. 2014). The respective data for median OS were 11.5 months for patients with 2 *TP53* alterations (2 hits) vs. not reached for patients with *TP53* deletion only ($P = .007$); vs. 63.1 months for cases with *TP53* mutation only ($P = .030$); vs. 60.2 months for *TP53* WT patients.

P53 Targeted Therapy

In normal unstressed cells, p53 is tightly regulated by MDM2/MDMX (MDM4) via ubiquitin/proteasome pathway. Reactivation of WT p53 function using MDM2/MDMX inhibitors in leukemic therapy has been investigated (Kojima, Ishizawa, and Andreeff 2016). MDM2 inhibition results in p53 stabilization and transcriptional activation of p53-target genes (Figure 3A, p53 targeted therapy). RG7112, a new member of the Nutlin family of MDM2 antagonists, prevents WT p53 from binding to its negative regulator of MDM2 (Fry et al. 2013). RG7112 was evaluated *in vitro* and *in vivo* by the Pediatric Preclinical Testing Program. RG7112 demonstrated sensitive cytotoxicity in 1 ALL cell line. Among 7 ALL xenografts, there was 1 PR, 5 CR, and 1 maintained CR (MCR) (Carol et al. 2013). As discussed earlier, in a phase 1 trial, RG7112 was administered to 116 patients (R/R AML, ALL, chronic myelogenous leukemia) and CLL/sCLL [small cell lymphocytic leukemia]). CR and PR were observed in 3 and 2 out of 30 evaluable AML patients (Andreeff et al. 2016). Clinical activity of RG7112 was also present in CLL/sCLL group. However, 3 evaluable ALL patients did not show response.

ETV6/RUNX1 (*E/R*) is the most common fusion gene in pediatric ALL. E/R was shown to upregulate MDM2 in primary ALL cells and cultured ALL cell lines. Inhibition of MDM2 using Nutlin-3a reactivated the p53 pathway in *E/R*-positive ALL leukemic cell lines and enhanced chemotherapy-induced apoptosis in *E/R*-positive primary leukemias (Kaindl et al. 2014). Effect of Nutlin-3a treatment was also evaluated in adult Philadelphia (Ph) positive ALL patients. Nutlin-3a reduced viability in Ph+, Ph- ALL cell lines and primary Ph+ leukemic cells. MDM2 inhibition activated p53 pathways in ALL cell lines with WT *TP53*, led to apoptosis and enhanced tyrosine kinase inhibitor-induced cell death (Trino, Iacobucci, et al. 2016).

MK8242 is another potent, orally bioavailable, small-molecule MDM2 inhibitor (Trino, De Luca, et al. 2016), which was evaluated in phase 1 clinical trial in solid tumors and R/R AML (Wagner et al. 2015, Ravandi et al. 2016). Kang et al. assessed its efficacy as a single agent *in vivo* and *in vitro* (Kang et al. 2016) and compared this study with their previous study of RG7112 in the same testing models (Carol et al. 2013). ALL cell lines were sensitive to MK8424 treatment. Among 10 ALL xenografts, 3 achieved CR or maintained CR (MCR) and 6 achieved PR. These results were comparable to RG7112 effect.

APR-246 was shown to restore WT conformation of p53 mutant protein and led to reactivation of p53 pathway and re-sensitization of *TP53* mutated (*TP53*mut) B-ALL cells or mice transplanted with *TP53*mut primograft to genotoxic therapy of doxorubicin (Demir et al. 2020). Reactivation of p53 pathway induced by APR-246 led to apoptosis. APR-246 strongly synergized with doxorubicin and re-sensitized *TP53*mut ALL to genotoxic therapy, which resulted in significantly increased survival compared to APR-246 alone ($P = 0.0005$).

TP53 ABERRATIONS IN B-CELL LYMPHOMAS

The frequency of *TP53* aberrations in B-cell lymphoma varies from 5% in extranodal marginal zone cell lymphoma with mucosa-associated lymphoid tissue (MALT) to 60% in B-cell prolymphocytic leukemia (B-PLL) (Tessoulin et al. 2017). *TP53* deletion is not detected in MALT. *TP53* deletion and *TP53* mutation occur in 5% and 15% B-ALL, respectively. In general, the prevalence of *TP53* aberration is in the range of 5-15% in low grade B-cell lymphomas in contrast to higher incidence of approximately 20-25% in more aggressive B-cell lymphomas such as BL, mantle cell lymphoma (MCL), and diffuse large B-cell lymphoma (DLBCL), especially in those derived from transformation of low-grade non-Hodgkin lymphoma (Cheung, Horsman, and Gascoyne 2009). There is no difference in incidence of *TP53* mutations in nodal vs. indolent leukemic variant of MCL (Sakhdari et al. 2019). *TP53* mutations occur in exons 5-9 (Peller and Rotter 2003, Cheung, Horsman, and Gascoyne 2009), the sequence-specific DNA-binding domain encompassing the highly conserved regions II–IV.

In addition to *TP53* aberration, p53 pathway is also impaired by dysregulations of its positive and negative regulators in B-cell lymphomas.

One of these mechanisms is MDM2 overexpression due to *mdm2* gene amplification, trisomy of chromosome 12 or downregulation of p53-induced miRNA192, 194, and 215. ARF inhibits MDM2 mediated proteolytic degradation of p53, which results in stabilization of p53 (Yu, Yu, and Young 2019). Loss of ARF leads to downregulation of p53 pathway.

Low frequency of MDM2 amplification occurs in low grade B-cell lymphomas including follicular lymphoma (FL), CLL/SLL, MALT, splenic marginal zone lymphoma, and lymphoplasmacytic lymphoma (Tessoulin et al. 2017). 10% of MCL show gain of *MDM2*, but 34% of them show MDM2 overexpression and majority of these MDM2 overexpressed cases are blastoid MCL (Solenthaler et al. 2002). Only 2% of BL and <1% DLBCL cases show *MDM2* amplification (Tessoulin et al. 2017). High incidence of loss of *ARF* mainly occurs in aggressive B-cell lymphomas such as B-ALL, MCL, and DLBCL whereas low frequency of this alteration is also present in BL and FL (Tessoulin et al. 2017).

Prognostic Impact of *TP53* Aberration in B-Cell Lymphomas

Chronic Lymphocytic Leukemia/Small Lymphocytic Lymphoma

Chronic lymphocytic leukemia/small lymphocytic lymphoma (CLL/SLL) is a B-cell lymphoproliferative disorder and the most common form of leukemia in adults (Nabhan and Rosen 2014). CLL/SLL is associated with a highly heterogeneous disease course, partially due to its diverse genetic alterations (Dohner et al. 2000, Landau et al. 2015, Baliakas et al. 2015). Generally, *TP53* aberration is associated with disease progression, poor treatment response, and inferior survival in B-cell lymphomas (Salmoiraghi, Rambaldi, and Spinelli 2018, Onaindia, Medeiros, and Patel 2017, Cheung, Horsman, and Gascoyne 2009, Voropaeva et al. 2019).

An international consortium of study groups has established *TP53* aberration (deletion or mutation) as one of five independent prognostic markers to further stratify patients into different subgroups using the data of 3472 treatment-naïve CLL/SLL patients from Europe and USA (Hallek

2017). Stengel et al. found that *TP53* aberration, mutation or deletion had an adverse impact on OS in the study with 1148 CLL/SLL patients (Stengel et al. 2017). Very high mutation loads (>75%) were also correlated to a worse OS (≤75% vs. >75%, not reached vs. 23 months, P = 0.007). A study through the European Research Initiative on chronic lymphocytic leukemia (ERIC) demonstrated *NOTCH1*, *SF3B1*, and *TP53* mutations were mostly enriched within clinically aggressive cases. (Baliakas et al. 2015). Likewise, *TP53* aberrations (deletion/mutation) correlated with a shorter time to first treatment (P < 0.0001) in 889 treatment-naive Binet stage A cases and retained independent significance in multivariate analysis.

TP53 aberration is associated with advanced stage, disease progression, and refractoriness to fludarabine regimen in CLL/SLL (Chiaretti et al. 2014, Xia et al. 2015, Onaindia, Medeiros, and Patel 2017). Rossi et al. showed that *TP53* mutations were associated with advanced Binet stage (P = 0.002), higher number of FISH lesions (P < 0.001), and occurrence of del17p13 (P < 0.001) (Rossi et al. 2009). *TP53* mutations predict inferior OS and chemoresistance to fludarabine based therapy independent of the concomitant occurrence of del17p13. Inactivation of the *TP53* is observed in approximately 60% of patients with Richter transformation (RS) and represents an independent predictor of OS after RS transformation (Rossi et al. 2011). Development of RS typically arises from the predominant CLL clone by acquiring an average of 20 genetic lesions/case. RS lesions are heterogeneous and include *TP53* disruption, *NOTCH* activation as well as some not previously implicated in CLL or RS pathogenesis (Fabbri et al. 2013).

Splenic Marginal Zone Lymphoma

Splenic marginal zone lymphoma (SMZL) is an indolent low-grade B-cell lymphoma involving the spleen and bone marrow characterized by a micronodular growth that replaces the preexisting lymphoid follicles and shows marginal zone differentiation (Piris, Onaindia, and Mollejo 2017). *TP53* deletion occurs in 3%-18% in SMZL (Salido et al. 2010, Piris, Onaindia, and Mollejo 2017). *TP53* mutations have been identified in 16% of SMZL (Parry et al. 2015). *TP53* and *NOTCH1* mutations are mutually exclusive (Jaramillo Oquendo et al. 2019). The presence of *TP53* deletions was an unfavorable indicator in a univariate analysis (median OS 5.6 vs. 11.6 years, $P < .035$). However, the prognostic significance was not retained in multivariate analysis (Salido et al. 2010). *TP53* mutations represented an independent prognostic factor for inferior OS. *TP53* mutated cases had a median OS of 12.2 years vs. 16.0 years for WT *TP53* cases (Parry et al. 2015).

Follicular Lymphoma

Follicular lymphoma (FL), the second most common type of non-Hodgkin lymphoma in the western world, is characterized by the t(14;18) translocation that is present in up to 90% of cases. *TP53* mutations and deletions are enriched in transformed FL compared to de novo FL (Bouska et al. 2014, Devan, Janikova, and Mraz 2018). *TP53* mutations are associated with early progression or transformation, older age, and high International Prognostic Index score in FL (Kridel et al. 2016, O' Shea et al. 2008). *TP53* deletions are associated with inferior PFS and OS in FL and their prognostic impact on OS is retained in multivariate analysis (Qu et al. 2019). On multivariate analysis, *TP53* mutation is associated with poor PFS ($P < .001$) and OS ($P = .009$) (O' Shea et al. 2008).

In addition, aberrations affecting TP53 regulators including MDM2 and MDM4 are even more frequent than *TP53* mutations (Devan, Janikova, and Mraz 2018). MDM2 overexpression was present in 72% of transformed FL compared to 58% of de novo FL (Davies et al. 2005). Amplification of *MDM2* and *MDM4* led to p53 degradation in 32% and 30% of transformed FL cases, in contrast to 23% and 17% of de novo FL, respectively (Bouska et al. 2014). Furthermore, p53 activity is impaired by aberrations affecting tumor suppressor genes such as *CDKN2A/B* (46% in transformed FL), whose protein products (p14-ARF, p16-INK4A and p15-INK4B) are critical as negative regulators of cell cycle G1 progression and as stabilizers of p53 (Pasqualucci et al. 2014).

Mantle Cell Lymphoma

Mantle cell lymphoma (MCL) is an aggressive mature B-cell non-Hodgkin lymphoma, which is defined by the t(11;14)(q13;q32) translocation which juxtaposes the *CCDN1* gene encoding cyclin D1 to the *immunoglobulin heavy chain (IgH)*, resulting in the overexpression of cyclin D1(Schieber, Gordon, and Karmali 2018). *TP53* mutations were shown to correlate with an inferior OS in MCL patients, as the median OS being13 months for *TP53* mutated cases vs. 43 months for cases with a WT *TP53* (Halldorsdottir et al. 2011). Interestingly, 17p deletions did not impact OS in the same cohort (median OS, 39 months vs. 35 months, respectively, $P = 0.7$). There was no correlation between *TP53* mutation and blastoid morphology in contrast to previous reports (Greiner et al. 1996, Hernandez et al. 1996). In a recent study, *TP53* mutation and deletion were significantly associated with poor Mantle Cell Lymphoma International Prognostic Index (MIPI), poor combined MIPI (MIPI-c), blastoid morphology, and Ki67 > 30%. *TP53*-mutated cases had a dismal clinical outcome, with a median OS of 1.8 years, and 50% relapsed at 1.0 years, compared to a median OS of 12.7 years for *TP53*-unmutated cases ($P < .0001$). Again, *TP53*-mutated cohorts also had inferior responses to both induction- and high-dose chemotherapy (Eskelund et al. 2017).

B-Cell Prolymphocytic Leukemia

B-cell prolymphocytic leukemia (B-PLL) is a rare disease, which accounts for < 1% chronic B-cell leukemia. A recent French study showed *TP53* mutation and *TP53* deletion were present in 38% of B-PLL cases, respectively (Chapiro et al. 2019). *MYC* aberration with rearrangement or gain was the most common cytogenetic abnormality, occurring in 76% of this cohort. These patients further stratified into three cytogenetic risk groups: low risk (no *MYC* aberration, median not reached; intermediate risk (*MYC* aberration but no *TP53* deletion, median OS: 125.7 months); high risk (both *MYC* aberration and *TP53* deletion, median OS: 11.1 months) (p=0.0006). Another early study also showed *TP53* mutation was detected in 38% of the B-PLL cases, which was associated with a dismal clinical outcome (Hercher et al. 2001). All six patients with mutant *TP53* died and 5 of them died within the first year of diagnosis.

Burkitt Lymphoma

Burkitt lymphoma (BL) is an aggressive B-cell lymphoma, which is defined by chromosomal translocation of *MYC* to *immunoglobulin heavy chain* or *light chain* and characterized by a high level of *MYC* expression. *TP53* is frequently mutated along several other genes including *MYC*, *ID3*, *ARID1A*, *SMAD4*, *PIK3R1*, and *NOTCH1* in BL (Love et al. 2012). *TP53* mutations were reported to be present in approximately 30% of adult BL cases (Gaidano et al. 1991), but only in 18% of pediatric BL (Leventaki et al. 2012). *TP53* deletion occurred in 10% of pediatric BL (Leventaki et al. 2012). In contrast, the frequency of p53 expression was much higher, which occurred in 50% of pediatric BL cohort (Leventaki et al. 2012). In the same study, TP53 negative regulators of MDM2 and MDM4 were also investigated. MDM4 overexpression, MDM2 overexpression, and gain of *MDM4* were present in 100%, 23%, and 21% of the cases, respectively. Cases with *MDM4* gain were correlated with cases lack of *TP53* aberration and p53 overexpression.

There are limited studies regarding prognostic impact of *TP53* mutation on BL. An early study form a Japanese group demonstrated that *TP53* mutation did not impact OS at 5 years while homozygous mutation of *TP53* did adversely impact OS at 5 years (Namiki et al. 2003). Another study showed BL patients had similar rate of CR, actuarial disease-free interval after 12 months, and actuarial survival rates after 24 months regardless of *TP53* mutation (Preudhomme et al. 1995).

Diffuse Large B-Cell Lymphoma

Diffuse large B-cell lymphoma (DLBCL), the most common non-Hodgkin lymphoma, accounts for one third of cases and is perhaps the most heterogeneous type of non-Hodgkin lymphoma. DLBCL has aggressive clinical features. The prevalence of *TP53* mutation and deletion is approximately 22% and 12.3% of DLBCL, respectively (Xu-Monette et al. 2012, Leroy et al. 2002, Cheung, Horsman, and Gascoyne 2009). Mutations of *TP53* are concentrated in exons 5-8 and majority of them occur in DNA-binding domain (Xu-Monette et al. 2012). Missense mutations comprise majority of the mutations, which are mainly LOF mutations.

TP53 mutation predicts poor survival in DLBCL patients, with a median OS of 94.49 months in WT *TP53* patients vs. 52.90 months in *TP53* mutated patients (Xu-Monette et al. 2012). The prognostic significance is also retained in DLBCL patients with germinal center type (GC) and DLBCL patients with activated B-cell like (ABC). In contrast, an earlier study showed *TP53* mutation adversely affected lymphoma-specific survival and progression survival in the entire DLBCL and GC-DLBCL patients, but not in non-GC DLBCL patients (Leroy et al. 2002). However, Xu-Monette et al. failed to show any prognostic impact of *TP53* deletion on survival (Xu-Monette et al. 2012). Additionally, p53 overexpression is frequent and associates with poor survival in DLBCL (Wang et al. 2017, Xie et al. 2014, Richardson, Zhang, et al. 2019). p53 expression further enhances negative impact of *MYC* rearrangement or MYC expression on OS in DLBCL exhibited in our recent study (Richardson, Zhang, et al. 2019).

Dysregulation of regulatory factors leads to dysfunction of p53 pathway in DLBCL. Copy number alteration (CNA) has decreased abundance of functional *TP53* and down-regulated levels of associated *TP53* targets (Lu et al. 2016). Copy loss of *CDKN2A*, at 9p21.3, occurs in 24% of DLBCLs. p16INK4A and p19ARF, these two alternative transcripts derived from the *CDKN2A* locus, play important roles in p53 signaling and cell cycle regulation. ARF interferes with binding of the MDM2 E3 ligase to p53, which attenuates MDM2 mediated p53 degradation (Brooks and Gu 2006). *MDM2* (12q15) amplification also occurs in 13% of the cohort. As a consequence, *CDKNA2* deletion (ARF loss) and *MDM2* (12q15) amplification both increase the ubiquitylation and subsequent degradation of p53 (Monti et al. 2012). *MDM4* amplification is present in 15% of cases, which can again result in inactivation of p53.

MDM2 amplification detected by fluorescence in situ hybridization (FISH) test is much lower, which was present in 0.3% of 364 DLBCL cases. However, MDM2 overexpression, defined by >10% cells positive for immunohistochemical staining, occurred in 40.4% of DLBCL cases in another study (Xu-Monette et al. 2013). MDM2 overexpression did not predict an adverse clinical outcome in patients with WT p53 but predicted significantly poorer survival in patients with mutated p53 in this study.

miRNAs are also key factors to control the normal p53 pathway, along with MDM2 and MDM4 which tightly regulate p53 activity under both normal and stressed conditions. miRNAs target the *TP53* directly or other components in the p53 signaling pathway so that expression and function of either the WT or the mutant forms of p53 is downregulated (Luo et al. 2018). The expression level of miR-34a is markedly decreased, which is associated with increased expression of FOXP1, p53, BCL-2, and poor OS in gastric DLBCL (He et al. 2014). The expression level of miR-34a is also lower in DLBCL cases carrying *TP53* deletion (Sun et al. 2013). DLBCL patients with combined *TP53* mutation and MIR34a methylation (double-hit) have an exceedingly poor prognosis with a median survival of 9.4 months ($p < 0.0001$) in comparison to patients with *TP53* mutation, MIR34A or MIR34B/C promoter methylation alone ("single hit") (Asmar et al. 2014).

P53 Targeted Therapy in B-Cell Lymphoma

Anti-Tumor Activity of Nutlin

Reactivation of p53, either by genetic manipulation or by application of small molecules that specifically target the p53 pathway, can result in the elimination of tumors mediated by induction of apoptosis. Nutlin-3a is a small molecule that activates the p53 pathway by disrupting p53-MDM2 interaction (Figure 3A, p53 targeted therapy). Drakos et al. demonstrated that Nutlin-3a activated p53 in DLBCL cells associated with t(14;18)(q32;q21) and WT p53 or in DLBCL cells with ABC cell of origin and WT p53. Activation of p53 pathway resulted in cell cycle arrest and apoptosis (Drakos et al. 2011). Nutlin-3a sensitized activation of the intrinsic apoptotic pathway induced by BCL2 inhibitors in t(14;18)-positive DLBCL cells with WT p53, and synergized doxorubicin cytotoxicity in t(14;18)-positive DLBCL cells carrying WT or mutant p53. Furthermore, Nutlin-3a treatment in xenograft animals inhibited lymphoma growth, accompanied by increased apoptosis and decreased proliferation. A recent study has shown that a novel BCL-2 inhibitor APG-2575 enhanced antitumor activity of Bruton Tyrosine Kinase inhibitor or MDM2-p53 inhibitor in DLBCL and prolonged survival in animal models (Luo et al. 2020).

Several studies have been performed to evaluate the impact of Nutlin on CLL/SLL. Nutlin-3a induced significant apoptosis in 30 (91%) of 33 samples from previously untreated patients with CLL; all resistant samples had *TP53* mutations. Nutlin-3a and Fludarabine, a chemotherapy agent, synergistically induced p53 and activated Bax, which resulted in activation of p53- mediated apoptotic pathway (Kojima et al. 2006). RG7388, a second generation of Nutlin family, decreased viability in CLL cells with WT *TP53*, but CLL cells with *TP53* aberrations were more resistant to the drug. RG7388 induced apoptosis by upregulating p53 target gene mediated intrinsic (*PUMA*, *BAX*) and extrinsic (*TNFRSF10B*, *FAS*) apoptotic pathways (Ciardullo et al. 2019). In a phase 1 trial, RG7112, a new member of Nutlin family, was administered to 116 patients (relapsed/refractory AML, ALL, chronic myelogenous leukemia) and CLL/sCLL [small cell lymphocytic leukemia]). CR and PR were observed in 10% and 7% of 30 evaluable AML patients (Andreeff et al. 2016). Clinical activity of RG7112 was also present in CLL/sCLL group. Of 19 evaluable CLL patients, 1 patient with CLL (history of prior Richter's transformation) had PR and continued on treatment for 25 cycles (NCT00623870).

Similar findings of anti-tumor effect of Nutlin-3a are also found in other B-cell and T-cell lymphomas. Nutlin-3a exerted anti-proliferative and proapoptotic activity and enhanced Bortezomib-mediated mitochondrial apoptosis in MCL cells (Tabe et al. 2009, Jin et al. 2010). Nutlin-3A increased p53 and induced cell cycle arrest and apoptosis in Hodgkin lymphoma, cutaneous T-cell lymphoma cell lines, adult T-cell leukemia cell lines, ALK+ anaplastic T-cell lymphoma, and BL cell lines (Drakos et al. 2007, Manfe et al. 2012, Hasegawa et al. 2009, Drakos et al. 2009).

Targeting p53 by RITA

Reactivation of p53 and induction of tumor cell apoptosis (RITA) is small molecule inhibitor, which disrupts binding of p53 and MDM2 (Figure

3A, p53 targeted therapy) (Cheok et al. 2011). RITA was initially reported to inhibit multiple myeloma (MM) cell growth via induction of p53-mediated apoptosis and synergistically enhanced Nutlin-induced cytotoxic response in MM cells (Saha, Jiang, Mukai, et al. 2010). One of molecular mechanisms of pro-apoptotic effect of RITA is activation of c-Jun N-terminal kinase (JNK) signaling pathway in MM (Saha et al. 2012). RITA was found to induce cell cycle arrest and apoptosis in MM and MCL cell lines resistant to MDM2 inhibitors MI-63 and Nutlin-3a. The drug resistance was mediated by acquired *TP53* mutations (Jones et al. 2012). Therefore, RITA can overcome TP53-mediated drug resistance probably by restoring WT p53 function. This proposed mechanism of RITA is also supported by the finding that RITA restores transcriptional transactivation and transrepression function of several hotspot p53 mutants (Zhao et al. 2010).

Restoration of Wild-Type Conformation of Mutant p53 by PRIMA-1

PRIMA-1 and PRIMA-1^{MET}(APR-246), methylated form of PRIMA, are a low-molecular weight compounds that can restore WT conformation of mutant p53 and sequence-specific DNA-binding and consequently triggers apoptosis in tumor cells carrying mutant p53 (Figure 3B, p53 targeted therapy). Apoptotic induction is mediated through restoration of the transcriptional transactivation function of mutant p53 (Bykov et al. 2002, Wiman 2010, Saha, Qiu, and Chang 2013). PRIMA-1 exerted cytotoxic effects on CLL/SLL cells from peripheral blood or bone marrows of patients with and without hemizygous *TP53* deletion. PRIMA-1 also exhibited synergistic and additive effects in combination with fludarabine (Nahi et al. 2004).

A recent study has also shown that PRIMA-1^{MET} was able to reduce mutated p53 protein in CLL cells, which was correlated with a significantly reduced viability and apoptosis induction (Jaskova et al. 2020). PRIMA-1^{MET}(APR-246) exerted antitumor activity by induction of p73 and Noxa in MM cell lines, delayed tumor growth, and prolonged survival of mice xenografted with MM tumor (Saha et al. 2013). PRIMA-1^{MET}(APR-246)-induced antitumor activity in MM cells was also mediated by demethylation of TP73, subsequently resulting in perturbation of endoplasmic reticulum

(ER) stress and deregulation of protein hemostasis. Cells without p53 expression demonstrated highest drug sensitivity (Teoh et al. 2016). These findings indicate apoptosis induced by PRIMA-1^{MET}(APR-246) can be p53 independent, which potentially extends therapeutic application of PRIMA-1^{MET}(APR-246) to a broader spectrum.

TP53 Aberrations in T-Cell Lymphomas

Peripheral T-cell lymphoma, not otherwise specified (PTCL, NOS), represents a clinically, histologically, and molecularly heterogeneous group of non-Hodgkin lymphomas. PTCLs exhibit an aggressive clinical course and are often refractory to standard therapy. Deletions of *TP53* and *9p21.3* containing *CDKN2A* encoding p16INK4A and p19ARF have occurred in 2 and 3 out 21 cases of PTCL, NOS, respectively (Vasmatzis et al. 2012). However, recent studies demonstrate that the distribution of *TP53* mutation and deletion and regulatory components of its pathway is likely related to different molecular profiles of PTCL. *TP53* aberrations are present in 16.5% of PTCL with T-follicular helper (TFH) cell phenotype and 23.2% of PTCL, NOS. More than half of *TP53* mutated/deleted PTCL, NOS are biallelic (Watatani et al. 2019). Aberration of *CDKN2A* (p14ARF), a MDM2 negative regulator, is more concentrated in PTCL, NOS, at a frequency of 12.8% in comparison of a frequency of 0.7% in PTCL-TFH (Watatani et al. 2019). Aberrations of *TP53* (58%) and *CDKN2A/2B* (p14ARF/p16INK4A) (45%) are also enriched in PTCL-GATA3 cases, a molecular subgroup of PTCL, NOS when compared to PTCL-TBX21 molecular subgroup (Heavican et al. 2019).

Anaplastic large cell lymphoma (ALCL) is a mature T-cell lymphoma with either a systemic, primary cutaneous, or breast implant presentation. Systemic ALCL represents a small subset of adult lymphomas (2%-5%), but up to 30% of pediatric cases. *TP53* deletion has occurred in 25% systemic ALCL, accounting for 9% of ALK+ALCL and 42% ALK-ALCL. Loss of *PRDM1*, a tumor suppressor gene, is frequently associated with loss of *TP53* and combined deletions of both genes predict an inferior clinical outcome (Boi et al. 2013).

TP53 mutations are rather infrequent in 8% of systemic ALCL whereas p53 expression is more common in 63% of ALCL patients (Rassidakis et al. 2005). Our study exhibits that p53 expression is associated with ALK-ALCL and poorer OS and DFS in patients with ALCL overall and in patients with ALK-ALCL (Richardson, Yin, et al. 2019). A recent study shows that *TP53* deletion is the most common cytogenetic aberration in all three types of ALCLs and fails to show any prognostic impact on clinical outcome (Gerbe et al. 2019).

Adult T-cell leukemia lymphoma (ATLL) is a rare T-cell leukemia caused by a retrovirus (human T-cell lymphotropic virus [HTLV]-1. ATLL is endemic in Japanese, Caribbean, and Latin American populations. Most North American ATLL patients are of Caribbean descent and are characterized by increased rate of chemoresistance and worse clinical outcome compared with Japanese ATLL (Shah et al. 2018). The incidence of *TP53* mutation is comparable in North American and Japanese ATLL cohorts, at 23% and 14%, respectively. *TP53*-mutated ATLL patients have a trend of worse OS ($p = 0.07$) (Shah et al. 2018).

T-cell prolymphocytic leukemia (T-PLL) is a rare and poor-prognostic mature T-cell malignancy. Somatic copy number alterations and mutations of *TP53* are rare, accounting for 4.8% (4/83 cases) and 3.7% (2/54 cases), respectively. In contrast, alterations of *TCL1A*, *ATM*, *AGO2*, or *MYC* are highly prevalent (Schrader et al. 2018).

Mycosis fungoides (MF) and Sezary syndrome (SS) are the most common cutaneous T-cell lymphomas and account for approximately 65% of cutaneous T-cell lymphomas. In the largest series of 101 SS cases studied so far (Woollard et al. 2016), *TP53* mutation or deletion was detected in only 15% and 6% of patients, respectively. Gros et al. found that *TP53* mutation and deletion occurred in 29% and 84% of primary and secondary SS cases, respectively (Gros et al. 2017). The *TP53* status did not provide prognostic significance. Patients with secondary SS had a worse prognosis than patients with primary SS.

TP53 ABERRATIONS IN MULTIPLE MYELOMA

Multiple myeloma (MM) is an incurable hematological malignancy developed as a result of clonal proliferation of plasma cells originating from fully differentiated B cells and represents the second most common hematological malignancy (Herrero et al. 2016). MM accounts for ~10% of all hematologic malignancies and affects elderly patients (Rajkumar 2016). MM is a clinically and biologically heterogenous disease characterized by a broad spectrum of genetic features including translocations, chromosomal copy number aberrations, and mutations in key oncogene and tumor suppressor genes (Morgan, Walker, and Davies 2012).

TP53 aberrations are relatively low in MM at diagnosis. *TP53* deletion is the most common abnormality at 8%, followed by mutation at 6%, and biallelic inactivation at 4% (Flynt et al. 2020, Walker et al. 2019). However, the incidence increases as the stage of disease advances, suggesting its essential role in disease progression. The incidence of *TP53* deletion in MM at relapse is in the range of 10% to 33% (Avet-Loiseau et al. 2017, Lakshman et al. 2019, Flynt et al. 2020). The frequency of *TP53* mutation in MM at relapse also increases to 25% (Kortum et al. 2016). The frequency of *TP53* aberrations (deletion and mutation) is much higher in more aggressive plasma cell neoplasm such as primary or secondary plasma cell leukemia, at 56% and 83%, respectively (Tiedemann et al. 2008). Analysis of co-occurrence of genomic events reveals that *TP53* mutations almost always occur after or simultaneously with *TP53* deletion (Chin et al. 2017). Inversely, *TP53* mutations are found in about one third of MM patients carrying *TP53* deletion, with the tendency of increase to more than 50% in refractory MM (Kortum et al. 2016, Lode et al. 2010).

TP53 aberrations continue to be important prognostic markers in MM. *TP53* deletion is one of the most powerful prognostic factors associated with an unfavorable outcome (Drach et al. 1998, Gutierrez et al. 2007, Fonseca et al. 2003). In an early study, patients with *TP53* deletion had significantly short OS compared to those without deletion, with a median OS of 13.9 months vs. 38.7 months (Drach et al. 1998). In multivariate analysis, *TP53* deletion also serves as an independent unfavorable prognostic marker

(Drach et al. 1998, Gutierrez et al. 2007). The prognostic significance of *TP53* deletion remains in relapsed MM receiving Lenalidomide Plus Dexamethasone, with a median time to progression of 2.2 months and a median OS of 4.67 months (Reece et al. 2009). *TP53* deletion is associated with extramedullary disease and refractoriness to chemotherapy (Deng et al. 2015, Lopez-Anglada et al. 2010). The clone size of *TP53* deletion also impacts the prognosis (An et al. 2015, Merz et al. 2016).

The presence of mutations in *TP53* is associated with an adverse outcome in terms of PFS and OS, while *TP53* deletion also predicts a shorter OS (Bolli et al. 2018). Study from Chin et al. found that *TP53* mutation was usually acquired after, or simultaneously with, allelic loss of 17p13, and conferred a significantly poorer prognosis for those patients with both abnormalities (Chin et al. 2017). At diagnosis, biallelic inactivation of *TP53* (double-hit MM) defines a subset of high-risk MM, which carries the poorest prognosis with a median PFS of 15.4 months and a median OS of 20.7 months (Walker et al. 2019). Likewise, biallelic *TP53* aberrations result in poorest prognosis at relapse (Weinhold et al. 2016).

MDM2, an important negative regulator of p53, is found to be deregulated in MM. MDM2 overexpression promotes proliferation and cell survival in MM cells. Inhibition of MDM2 leads to cell apoptosis (Teoh et al. 1997). Upregulation of MDM2 mRNA was reported in 2 out of 4 MMs (Quesnel et al. 1994). MDM2 amplification was identified in 8%, while another 8% had trisomy 12 with an equivalent increase in signals for MDM2 in a series of 82 MM cohort (Elnenaei et al. 2003). High level of MDM2 overexpression is associated with a poor clinical outcome (Teoh et al. 2014).

Deregulation of miRNAs in cancer is being rigorously explored and has led to the investigation of the role of miRNAs in the pathogenesis of MM (Handa et al. 2019). The first evidence of the involvement of miRNA in MM pathogenesis demonstrates that MM cell lines and MM samples display a reduced expression of miR-125b, miR-133a, miR-1, miR-124a, miR-15, and miR-16 than their normal counterparts (Al-Masri et al. 2005). Distinct expression patterns of miR-21, miR-106b, miR-181a and b, miR-32, and miR-17 between monoclonal gammopathy of undetermined significance (MGUS) and MM plasma cells and normal plasma cells also suggest a role of miRNAs in MM neoplastic transformation and progression (Pichiorri et al. 2008). Studies on the miRNA regulation on p53 expression have identified that both miRNA-25 and miRNA-30d directly targeted the 3'-UTR of p53 mRNA and subsequently resulted in decrease of p53 protein expression, depletion of the apoptosis response rate, and decline of cellular senescence in several cell lines. Downregulation of these two miRNAs increases p53 expression and results in increased apoptosis in MM cell line (Kumar et al. 2011). miR-192, 194, and 215 are also found to be downregulated in a subset of MMs and are amenable to transcriptional activation by p53. Ectopic expression of miR-192, 194, and 215 leads to increased expression of p53 and sensitizes MDM2 inhibitor-induced apoptosis in MM cell line and MM cell-engrafted mice (Pichiorri et al. 2010).

In MM, altered expression of miRNAs is found to be associated with chromosomal abnormalities. Differential miRNA expression patterns are mainly associated with the major *IGH* translocations; particularly, t(4;14) patients exhibit specific overexpression of let-7e, miR-125a-5p, and miR-99b in purified MM cells (Lionetti 2009). miR-15a/16 cluster and miR-17-92 cluster (miR-17, miR19a, and miR-20a) are downregulated in primary MM samples with del13q (Handa et al. 2019). Similarly, miR-22, encoded at the 17p locus, is significantly under-expressed in those patients with the 17p deletion (Lionetti et al. 2009).

Although miRNA expression is often downregulated in many cancers including MM, the overall underlying mechanism is not yet fully understood. It has recently been shown that miRNA expression is itself epigenetically regulated by methylation and histone acetylation (Handa et al. 2019). miR-34a/b/c, miR-124-1, miR-194-2, miR-192, miR-203, miR-152, and miR-10b-5p have been reported to be frequently methylated in MM (Handa et al. 2019). The target genes of these miRNAs are responsible for cell survival, proliferation, anti-apoptosis, and drug resistance (Misiewicz-Krzeminska et al. 2019, Handa et al. 2019). For example, hypermethylation-dependent inhibition of miR-152, -10b-5p, and -34c-3p indicates their putative tumor suppressor role in MM. Demethylation or gain of function studies of these specific miRNAs has resulted in apoptosis, reduced proliferation, and down-regulation of putative oncogene targets of these miRNAs such as *DNMT1*, *E2F3*, *BTRC*, and *MYCBP* (Zhang et al. 2014).

miRNAs are also regulated by other epigenetic mechanisms such as histone modification (Handa et al. 2019). Silencing of histone deacetylase 4 (HDAC4) by short hairpin RNAs results in hyperacetylation of miR-29-a/b1 promoter, increased miR-29b expression, and downregulation of miR-29b pro-survival targets (*SP1* and *MCL-1*). The ultimate outcomes of downregulated pro-survival lead to reduced cell survival and migration and induction of apoptosis and autophagy in MM. Treatment with the pan-HDAC inhibitor SAHA also upregulates miR-29b and results in inhibition of cell growth and induction of apoptosis and autophagy (Amodio et al. 2016).

P53 Targeted Therapy

Proteasome Inhibitors

Bortezomib was approved by the Food and Drug Administration (FDA) for MM treatment in 2008. Bortezomib is a proteasome inhibitor. It has a potent anti-myeloma activity both when used as a single agent and in combination with other drugs (Castelli et al. 2013). 26S proteasome is a large protein complex responsible for degradation of intracellular proteins that have been polyubiquitinated by E1, E2, and E3 ubiquitin ligases (Tanaka 2009). MDM2 is an E3 ubiquitin ligase that facilitates the p53 ubiquitination and subsequently induces its proteolytic degradation in the 26S proteasome complex, therefore keeping p53 expression under control at normal conditions. In MM, overexpression of MDM2 elicits increased proteasomal degradation of p53 (Teoh and Chng 2014). Therefore, bortezomib exerts its effects by blocking the turnover of poly-ubiquitinated proteins through the proteasome, thus preventing p53 from being degraded (Figure 3C, p53 targeted therapy) (Hideshima et al. 2003).

Inhibitors of p53-MDM2 Interaction

As we discussed in previous sections, Nutlin-3a is a small molecule that activates the p53 pathway by disrupting p53-MDM2 interaction (Figure 3A, p53 targeted therapy). Saha et al. found that Nutlin-induced apoptosis correlated with reduction in cell viability, upregulation of p53, p21, and proapoptotic targets MDM2, PUMA, Bax, and Bak, downregulation of anti-apoptotic targets BCL2 and survivin, and activation of caspase in MM cell lines with WT *TP53* (Figure 3A, p53 targeted therapy) (Saha, Jiang, and Chang 2010). In addition, combined treatment with Nutlin and Velcade, a proteasome inhibitor, shows synergic antimyeloma activity evidenced by decrease in cell viability, increased expression of p53, MDM2, p21, as well as caspase activation and induction of proapoptotic targets in MM cells (Saha, Jiang, Jayakar, et al. 2010).

RITA is small molecule inhibitor, which disrupts binding of p53 and MDM2 (Figure 3A, p53 targeted therapy) (Cheok et al. 2011). As we discussed in previous section, RITA was initially reported to inhibit MM cell growth via p53-mediated apoptosis and cooperatively enhanced Nutlin-induced cytotoxic response in MM cells (Saha, Jiang, Mukai, et al. 2010). Subsequently, RITA-induced apoptosis in MM cells was also found to mediate through activation of JNK signaling pathway and p53 independent pathway (Saha et al. 2012, Surget et al. 2014).

AMG 232 is an investigational oral, selective inhibitor of the MDM2-p53 protein-protein interaction (Figure 3A, p53 targeted therapy) (Sun et al. 2014). AMG 232 inhibits *in vivo* growth of several tumor xenografts via p53-mediated induction of apoptosis (Canon et al. 2015). A recent study also reveals glioblastoma stem cells are highly susceptible to AMG 232 treatment (Her et al. 2018). In a phase 1 multicenter clinical trial, AMG 232 as monotherapy administered to patients with p53 WT advanced solid tumors or MM displayed acceptable safety and dose-proportional pharmacokinetics, and stable disease was observed (Gluck et al. 2020).

USP7, one of the most studied deubiquitinating enzymes, is critical in protecting MDM2 and MDMX (MDM4) from ubiquitination-mediated proteasomal degradation. USP7 inhibition leads to the degradation of MDM2 and MDMX and activation of p53 signaling pathway (Qi et al.

2020). USP7 inhibitor induces apoptosis by promoting MDM2 degradation that increases p53 and p21 expression in MM cell lines (Figure 3C, p53 targeted therapy). In addition, USP7 inhibitor also overcomes bortezomib-resistance and displays synergistic anti-MM activity with lenalidomide, dexamethasone or the HDAC inhibitor (Chauhan et al. 2012).

Targeting Mutant p53

Discovery of small molecules or peptides that stabilize mutant p53 in biologic conformation, restore its DNA-binding ability and thus rescue its WT activity becomes a pressing issue. PRIMA-1 is a small molecule drug that rescues mutant p53 by restoring its active conformation and transcriptional functions, consequently triggering massive apoptosis in tumor cells carrying mutant p53 (Figure 3B, p53 targeted therapy). PRIMA-1^{MET}(APR-246) exerts antitumor activity irrespective of their p53 status. This cytotoxic effect is mediated by induction of p73 and Noxa in MM cell lines and mice xenografted with MM tumor (Saha et al. 2013). Teoh et al. confirmed this novel p53-independent mechanism of PRIMA-1^{MET} induced antitumor activity and p73 activation in MM cells was mediated by demethylation of *TP73* (Teoh et al. 2016). PRIMA-1^{MET} induced antimyeloma activity was also mediated by impairing oxidative stress pathway (Tessoulin et al. 2019, Tessoulin et al. 2014).

MIRA-1, a novel class of mutant p53 reactivating molecules, which is structurally distinct from PRIMA-1, was identified in the similar screening by the same groups (Figure 3B, p53 targeted therapy) (Bykov et al. 2005). MIRA-1 treatment results in inhibition of viability, colony formation and migration, and increase in apoptosis of MM cells irrespective of p53 status. MIRA-1 also reduces tumor burden in MM xenograft mice. Lastly, combined treatment of MIRA-1 with dexamethasone, doxorubicin or Velcade displays synergistic effect in MM cells and mice bearing MM tumor (Saha et al. 2014).

CONCLUSION

TP53 aberrations are of poor prognosis and indicative of disease progression in hematologic malignancies. This review focuses on the incidence of *TP53* aberrations and molecular mechanisms of *TP53* dysregulation, such as 17p deletion, *TP53* mutations, p53 overexpression, MDM2 and MDM4 overexpression, downregulation of ARF, methylation of *TP53* promoter, and deregulation of miRNAs in hematologic neoplasms. Understanding these regulatory mechanisms of p53 signaling pathway has facilitated the development of therapeutic agents to specifically target each component of this pathway. Different strategies are currently engaged: blocking the interaction between MDM2 and p53 with small molecules such as Nutlin, RITA, ALRN-6924, targeting MDM2 by blocking its deubiquitination by USP7 inhibitors, reduction of p53 degradation by proteasome inhibitor, and rescuing the function of mutant p53 proteins with small molecules such as PRIMA-1 and MIRA-1. All these therapeutic strategies have been evaluated *in vitro* and *in vivo* and some of these therapies have advanced to clinical trials.

ACKNOWLEDGMENTS

I want to thank Ms. Sonora Thigpen for her editorial work on the manuscript and assistance of the figures.

REFERENCES

Al-Masri, A., Price-Troska, T., Chesi, M., Chung, T. H., Kim, S., Carpten, J., Bergsagel, P. L. & Fonseca, R. (2005). "MicroRNA Expression Analysis in Multiple Myeloma." *Blood., 106*, 1554.

Amodio, N., Stamato, M. A., Gulla, A. M., Morelli, E., Romeo, E., Raimondi, L., Pitari, M. R., Ferrandino, I., Misso, G., Caraglia, M., Perrotta, I., Neri, A., Fulciniti, M., Rolfo, C., Anderson, K. C., Munshi,

N. C., Tagliaferri, P. & Tassone, P. (2016). "Therapeutic Targeting of miR-29b/HDAC4 Epigenetic Loop in Multiple Myeloma." *Mol Cancer Ther*, *15* (6), 1364-75. doi: 10.1158/1535-7163.MCT-15-0985.

An, G., Li, Z., Tai, Y. T., Acharya, C., Li, Q., Qin, X., Yi, S., Xu, Y., Feng, X., Li, C., Zhao, J., Shi, L., Zang, M., Deng, S., Sui, W., Hao, M., Zou, D., Zhao, Y., Qi, J., Cheng, T., Ru, K., Wang, J., Anderson, K. C. & Qiu, L. (2015). "The impact of clone size on the prognostic value of chromosome aberrations by fluorescence *in situ* hybridization in multiple myeloma." *Clin Cancer Res*, *21* (9), 2148-56. doi: 10.1158/1078-0432.CCR-14-2576.

Andreeff, M., Kelly, K. R., Yee, K., Assouline, S., Strair, R., Popplewell, L., Bowen, D., Martinelli, G., Drummond, M. W., Vyas, P., Kirschbaum, M., Iyer, S. P., Ruvolo, V., Gonzalez, G. M., Huang, X., Chen, G., Graves, B., Blotner, S., Bridge, P., Jukofsky, L., Middleton, S., Reckner, M., Rueger, R., Zhi, J., Nichols, G. & Kojima, K. (2016). "Results of the Phase I Trial of RG7112, a Small-Molecule MDM2 Antagonist in Leukemia." *Clin Cancer Res*, *22* (4), 868-76. doi: 10.1158/1078-0432.CCR-15-0481.

Argiropoulos, B. & Humphries, R. K. (2007). "Hox genes in hematopoiesis and leukemogenesis." *Oncogene*, *26* (47), 6766-76. doi: 10.1038/sj.onc.1210760.

Asmar, F., Hother, C., Kulosman, G., Treppendahl, M. B., Nielsen, H. M., Ralfkiaer, U., Pedersen, A., Moller, M. B., Ralfkiaer, E., de Nully Brown, P. & Gronbaek, K. (2014). "Diffuse large B-cell lymphoma with combined TP53 mutation and MIR34A methylation: Another "double hit" lymphoma with very poor outcome?" *Oncotarget*, *5* (7), 1912-25. doi: 10.18632/oncotarget.1877.

Avet-Loiseau, H., Bahlis, N. J., Chng, W. J., Masszi, T., Viterbo, L., Pour, L., Ganly, P., Palumbo, A., Cavo, M., Langer, C., Pluta, A., Nagler, A., Kumar, S., Ben-Yehuda, D., Rajkumar, S. V., San-Miguel, J., Berg, D., Lin, J., van de Velde, H., Esseltine, D. L., di Bacco, A., Moreau, P. & Richardson, P. G. (2017). "Ixazomib significantly prolongs progression-free survival in high-risk relapsed/refractory myeloma patients." *Blood*, *130* (24), 2610-2618. doi: 10.1182/blood-2017-06-791228.

Baliakas, P., Hadzidimitriou, A., Sutton, L. A., Rossi, D., Minga, E., Villamor, N., Larrayoz, M., Kminkova, J., Agathangelidis, A., Davis, Z., Tausch, E., Stalika, E., Kantorova, B., Mansouri, L., Scarfo, L., Cortese, D., Navrkalova, V., Rose-Zerilli, M. J., Smedby, K. E., Juliusson, G., Anagnostopoulos, A., Makris, A. M., Navarro, A., Delgado, J., Oscier, D., Belessi, C., Stilgenbauer, S., Ghia, P., Pospisilova, S., Gaidano, G., Campo, E., Strefford, J. C., Stamatopoulos, K., Rosenquist, R. & European Research Initiative on, C. L. L. (2015). "Recurrent mutations refine prognosis in chronic lymphocytic leukemia." *Leukemia*, *29* (2), 329-36. doi: 10.1038/leu.2014.196.

Barbosa, K., Li, S., Adams, P. D. & Deshpande, A. J. (2019). "The role of TP53 in acute myeloid leukemia: Challenges and opportunities." *Genes Chromosomes Cancer*, *58* (12), 875-888. doi: 10.1002/ gcc.22796.

Boi, M., Rinaldi, A., Kwee, I., Bonetti, P., Todaro, M., Tabbo, F., Piva, R., Rancoita, P. M., Matolcsy, A., Timar, B., Tousseyn, T., Rodriguez-Pinilla, S. M., Piris, M. A., Bea, S., Campo, E., Bhagat, G., Swerdlow, S. H., Rosenwald, A., Ponzoni, M., Young, K. H., Piccaluga, P. P., Dummer, R., Pileri, S., Zucca, E., Inghirami, G. & Bertoni, F. (2013). "PRDM1/BLIMP1 is commonly inactivated in anaplastic large T-cell lymphoma." *Blood*, *122* (15), 2683-93. doi: 10.1182/blood-2013-04-497933.

Bolli, N., Biancon, G., Moarii, M., Gimondi, S., Li, Y., de Philippis, C., Maura, F., Sathiaseelan, V., Tai, Y. T., Mudie, L., O' Meara, S., Raine, K., Teague, J. W., Butler, A. P., Carniti, C., Gerstung, M., Bagratuni, T., Kastritis, E., Dimopoulos, M., Corradini, P., Anderson, K. C., Moreau, P., Minvielle, S., Campbell, P. J., Papaemmanuil, E., Avet-Loiseau, H. & Munshi, N. C. (2018). "Analysis of the genomic landscape of multiple myeloma highlights novel prognostic markers and disease subgroups." *Leukemia*, *32* (12), 2604-2616. doi: 10.1038/s41375-018-0037-9.

Bouska, A., McKeithan, T. W., Deffenbacher, K. E., Lachel, C., Wright, G. W., Iqbal, J., Smith, L. M., Zhang, W., Kucuk, C., Rinaldi, A., Bertoni, F., Fitzgibbon, J., Fu, K., Weisenburger, D. D., Greiner, T. C., Dave, B. J., Gascoyne, R. D., Rosenwald, A., Ott, G., Campo, E., Rimsza, L. M., Delabie, J., Jaffe, E. S., Braziel, R. M., Connors, J. M., Staudt, L. M. &

Chan, W. C. (2014). "Genome-wide copy-number analyses reveal genomic abnormalities involved in transformation of follicular lymphoma." *Blood*, *123* (11), 1681-90. doi: 10.1182/blood-2013-05-500595.

Brooks, C. L. & Gu, W. (2006). "p53 ubiquitination: Mdm2 and beyond." *Mol Cell*, *21* (3), 307-15. doi: 10.1016/j.molcel.2006.01.020.

Bueso-Ramos, C. E., Manshouri, T., Haidar, M. A., Huh, Y. O., Keating, M. J. & Albitar, M. (1995). "Multiple patterns of MDM-2 deregulation in human leukemias: implications in leukemogenesis and prognosis." *Leuk Lymphoma*, *17* (1-2), 13-8. doi: 10.3109/10428199509051698.

Bueso-Ramos, C. E., Yang, Y., deLeon, E., McCown, P., Stass, S. A. & Albitar, M. (1993). "The human MDM-2 oncogene is overexpressed in leukemias." *Blood*, *82* (9), 2617-23.

Bykov, V. J., Issaeva, N., Shilov, A., Hultcrantz, M., Pugacheva, E., Chumakov, P., Bergman, J., Wiman, K. G. & Selivanova, G. (2002). "Restoration of the tumor suppressor function to mutant p53 by a low-molecular-weight compound." *Nat Med*, *8* (3), 282-8. doi: 10.1038/nm0302-282.

Bykov, V. J., Issaeva, N., Zache, N., Shilov, A., Hultcrantz, M., Bergman, J., Selivanova, G. & Wiman, K. G. (2005). "Reactivation of mutant p53 and induction of apoptosis in human tumor cells by maleimide analogs." *J Biol Chem*, *280* (34), 30384-91. doi: 10.1074/jbc.M501664200.

Canon, J., Osgood, T., Olson, S. H., Saiki, A. Y., Robertson, R., Yu, D., Eksterowicz, J., Ye, Q., Jin, L., Chen, A., Zhou, J., Cordover, D., Kaufman, S., Kendall, R., Oliner, J. D., Coxon, A. & Radinsky, R. (2015). "The MDM2 Inhibitor AMG 232 Demonstrates Robust Antitumor Efficacy and Potentiates the Activity of p53-Inducing Cytotoxic Agents." *Mol Cancer Ther*, *14* (3), 649-58. doi: 10.1158/1535-7163.MCT-14-0710.

Carol, H., Reynolds, C. P., Kang, M. H., Keir, S. T., Maris, J. M., Gorlick, R., Kolb, E. A., Billups, C. A., Geier, B., Kurmasheva, R. T., Houghton, P. J., Smith, M. A. & Lock, R. B. (2013). "Initial testing of the MDM2 inhibitor RG7112 by the Pediatric Preclinical Testing Program." *Pediatr Blood Cancer*, *60* (4), 633-41. doi: 10.1002/pbc.24235.

Carvajal, L. A., Neriah, D. B., Senecal, A., Benard, L., Thiruthuvanathan, V., Yatsenko, T., Narayanagari, S. R., Wheat, J. C., Todorova, T. I., Mitchell, K., Kenworthy, C., Guerlavais, V., Annis, D. A., Bartholdy, B., Will, B., Anampa, J. D., Mantzaris, I., Aivado, M., Singer, R. H., Coleman, R. A., Verma, A. & Steidl, U. (2018). "Dual inhibition of MDMX and MDM2 as a therapeutic strategy in leukemia." *Sci Transl Med*, *10* (436). doi: 10.1126/scitranslmed.aao3003.

Cassier, P. A., Castets, M., Belhabri, A. & Vey, N. (2017). "Targeting apoptosis in acute myeloid leukaemia." *Br J Cancer*, *117* (8), 1089-1098. doi: 10.1038/bjc.2017.281.

Castelli, R., Gualtierotti, R., Orofino, N., Losurdo, A., Gandolfi, S. & Cugno, M. (2013). "Current and emerging treatment options for patients with relapsed myeloma." *Clin Med Insights Oncol*, *7*, 209-19. doi: 10.4137/CMO.S8014.

Chapiro, E., Pramil, E., Diop, M., Roos-Weil, D., Dillard, C., Gabillaud, C., Maloum, K., Settegrana, C., Baseggio, L., Lesesve, J. F., Yon, M., Jondreville, L., Lesty, C., Davi, F., Le Garff-Tavernier, M., Droin, N., Dessen, P., Algrin, C., Leblond, V., Gabarre, J., Bouzy, S., Eclache, V., Gaillard, B., Callet-Bauchu, E., Muller, M., Lefebvre, C., Nadal, N., Ittel, A., Struski, S., Collonge-Rame, M. A., Quilichini, B., Fert-Ferrer, S., Auger, N., Radford-Weiss, I., Wagner, L., Scheinost, S., Zenz, T., Susin, S. A., Bernard, O. A., Nguyen-Khac, F. & Hematologique the Groupe Francophone de Cytogenetique, and Organization the French Innovative Leukemia. (2019). "Genetic characterization of B-cell prolymphocytic leukemia: a prognostic model involving MYC and TP53." *Blood*, *134* (21), 1821-1831. doi: 10.1182/blood.2019001187.

Chauhan, D., Tian, Z., Nicholson, B., Kumar, K. G., Zhou, B., Carrasco, R., McDermott, J. L., Leach, C. A., Fulciniti, M., Kodrasov, M. P., Weinstock, J., Kingsbury, W. D., Hideshima, T., Shah, P. K., Minvielle, S., Altun, M., Kessler, B. M., Orlowski, R., Richardson, P., Munshi, N. & Anderson, K. C. (2012). "A small molecule inhibitor of ubiquitin-specific protease-7 induces apoptosis in multiple myeloma cells and overcomes bortezomib resistance." *Cancer Cell*, *22* (3), 345-58. doi: 10.1016/j.ccr.2012.08.007.

Cheok, C. F., Verma, C. S., Baselga, J. & Lane, D. P. (2011). "Translating p53 into the clinic." *Nat Rev Clin Oncol*, *8* (1), 25-37. doi: 10.1038/nrclinonc.2010.174.

Cheung, K. J., Horsman, D. E. & Gascoyne, R. D. (2009). "The significance of TP53 in lymphoid malignancies: mutation prevalence, regulation, prognostic impact and potential as a therapeutic target." *Br J Haematol*, *146* (3), 257-69. doi: 10.1111/j.1365-2141.2009.07739.x.

Chiaretti, S., Brugnoletti, F., Tavolaro, S., Bonina, S., Paoloni, F., Marinelli, M., Patten, N., Bonifacio, M., Kropp, M. G., Sica, S., Guarini, A. & Foa, R. (2013). "TP53 mutations are frequent in adult acute lymphoblastic leukemia cases negative for recurrent fusion genes and correlate with poor response to induction therapy." *Haematologica*, *98* (5), e59-61. doi: 10.3324/haematol.2012.076786.

Chiaretti, S., Marinelli, M., Del Giudice, I., Bonina, S., Piciocchi, A., Messina, M., Vignetti, M., Rossi, D., Di Maio, V., Mauro, F. R., Guarini, A., Gaidano, G. & Foa, R. (2014). "NOTCH1, SF3B1, BIRC3 and TP53 mutations in patients with chronic lymphocytic leukemia undergoing first-line treatment: correlation with biological parameters and response to treatment." *Leuk Lymphoma*, *55* (12), 2785-92. doi: 10.3109/10428194.2014.898760.

Chin, M., Sive, J. I., Allen, C., Roddie, C., Chavda, S. J., Smith, D., Blombery, P., Jones, K., Ryland, G. L., Popat, R., Rismani, A., D'Sa, S., Rabin, N., Gale, R. E. & Yong, K. L. (2017). "Prevalence and timing of TP53 mutations in del(17p) myeloma and effect on survival." *Blood Cancer J*, *7* (9), e610. doi: 10.1038/bcj.2017.76.

Ciardullo, C., Aptullahoglu, E., Woodhouse, L., Lin, W. Y., Wallis, J. P., Marr, H., Marshall, S., Bown, N., Willmore, E. & Lunec, J. (2019). "Non-genotoxic MDM2 inhibition selectively induces a pro-apoptotic p53 gene signature in chronic lymphocytic leukemia cells." *Haematologica*, *104* (12), 2429-2442. doi: 10.3324/haematol.2018.206631.

Cluzeau, T., Sebert, M., Rahmé, R., Cuzzubbo, S., Walter-petrich, A., Lehmann che, J., Peterlin, P., Beve, B., Attalah, H., Chermat, F., Miekoutima, E., Beyne-Rauzy, O., Recher, C., Stamatoullas, A.,

Willems, L., Raffoux, E., Berthon, C., Quesnel, B., Carpentier, A., Sallman, D. A., Chevret, S., Ades, L. & Fenaux, P. (2019). "APR-246 Combined with Azacitidine (AZA) in TP53 Mutated Myelodysplastic Syndrome (MDS) and Acute Myeloid Leukemia (AML). a Phase 2 Study By the Groupe Francophone Des Myélodysplasies (GFM)." *Blood*. doi: https://doi.org/10.1182/blood-2019-125579.

Colombo, E., Martinelli, P., Zamponi, R., Shing, D. C., Bonetti, P., Luzi, L., Volorio, S., Bernard, L., Pruneri, G., Alcalay, M. & Pelicci, P. G. (2006). "Delocalization and destabilization of the Arf tumor suppressor by the leukemia-associated NPM mutant." *Cancer Res*, 66 (6), 3044-50. doi: 10.1158/0008-5472.CAN-05-2378.

Cumbo, C., Tota, G., Anelli, L., Zagaria, A., Specchia, G. & Albano, F. (2020). "TP53 in Myelodysplastic Syndromes: Recent Biological and Clinical Findings." *Int J Mol Sci*, 21 (10). doi: 10.3390/ijms21103432.

Davies, A. J., Lee, A. M., Taylor, C., Clear, A. J., Goff, L. K., Iqbal, S., Cuthbert-Heavens, D., Calaminici, M., Norton, A. J., Lister, T. A. & Fitzgibbon, J. (2005). "A limited role for TP53 mutation in the transformation of follicular lymphoma to diffuse large B-cell lymphoma." *Leukemia*, 19 (8), 1459-65. doi: 10.1038/sj.leu.2403802.

Demir, S., Boldrin, E., Sun, Q., Hampp, S., Tausch, E., Eckert, C., Ebinger, M., Handgretinger, R., Kronnie, G. T., Wiesmuller, L., Stilgenbauer, S., Selivanova, G., Debatin, K. M. & Meyer, L. H. (2020). "Therapeutic targeting of mutant p53 in pediatric acute lymphoblastic leukemia." *Haematologica*, 105 (1), 170-181. doi: 10.3324/haematol.2018.199364.

Deng, S., Xu, Y., An, G., Sui, W., Zou, D., Zhao, Y., Qi, J., Li, F., Hao, M. & Qiu, L. (2015). "Features of extramedullary disease of multiple myeloma: high frequency of p53 deletion and poor survival: a retrospective single-center study of 834 cases." *Clin Lymphoma Myeloma Leuk*, 15 (5), 286-91. doi: 10.1016/j.clml.2014.12.013.

Devan, J., Janikova, A. & Mraz, M. (2018). "New concepts in follicular lymphoma biology: From BCL2 to epigenetic regulators and non-coding RNAs." *Semin Oncol*, 45 (5-6), 291-302. doi: 10.1053/j.seminoncol.2018.07.005.

Ding, Q., Zhang, Z., Liu, J. J., Jiang, N., Zhang, J., Ross, T. M., Chu, X. J., Bartkovitz, D., Podlaski, F., Janson, C., Tovar, C., Filipovic, Z. M., Higgins, B., Glenn, K., Packman, K., Vassilev, L. T. & Graves, B. (2013). "Discovery of RG7388, a potent and selective p53-MDM2 inhibitor in clinical development." *J Med Chem, 56* (14), 5979-83. doi: 10.1021/jm400487c.

Dohner, H., Dolnik, A., Tang, L., Seymour, J. F., Minden, M. D., Stone, R. M., Del Castillo, T. B., Al-Ali, H. K., Santini, V., Vyas, P., Beach, C. L., MacBeth, K. J., Skikne, B. S., Songer, S., Tu, N., Bullinger, L. & Dombret, H. (2018). "Cytogenetics and gene mutations influence survival in older patients with acute myeloid leukemia treated with azacitidine or conventional care." *Leukemia, 32* (12), 2546-2557. doi: 10.1038/s41375-018-0257-z.

Dohner, H., Stilgenbauer, S., Benner, A., Leupolt, E., Krober, A., Bullinger, L., Dohner, K., Bentz, M. & Lichter, P. (2000). "Genomic aberrations and survival in chronic lymphocytic leukemia." *N Engl J Med, 343* (26), 1910-6. doi: 10.1056/NEJM200012283432602.

Drach, J., Ackermann, J., Fritz, E., Kromer, E., Schuster, R., Gisslinger, H., DeSantis, M., Zojer, N., Fiegl, M., Roka, S., Schuster, J., Heinz, R., Ludwig, H. & Huber, H. (1998). "Presence of a p53 gene deletion in patients with multiple myeloma predicts for short survival after conventional-dose chemotherapy." *Blood, 92* (3), 802-9.

Drakos, E., Atsaves, V., Schlette, E., Li, J., Papanastasi, I., Rassidakis, G. Z. & Medeiros, L. J. (2009). "The therapeutic potential of p53 reactivation by nutlin-3a in ALK+ anaplastic large cell lymphoma with wild-type or mutated p53." *Leukemia, 23* (12), 2290-9. doi: 10.1038/leu.2009.180.

Drakos, E., Singh, R. R., Rassidakis, G. Z., Schlette, E., Li, J., Claret, F. X., Ford, R. J., Jr. Vega, F. & Medeiros, L. J. (2011). "Activation of the p53 pathway by the MDM2 inhibitor nutlin-3a overcomes BCL2 overexpression in a preclinical model of diffuse large B-cell lymphoma associated with t(14;18)(q32;q21)." *Leukemia, 25* (5), 856-67. doi: 10.1038/leu.2011.28.

Drakos, E., Thomaides, A., Medeiros, L. J., Li, J., Leventaki, V., Konopleva, M., Andreeff, M. & Rassidakis, G. Z. (2007). "Inhibition of p53-murine double minute 2 interaction by nutlin-3A stabilizes p53 and induces cell cycle arrest and apoptosis in Hodgkin lymphoma." *Clin Cancer Res*, *13* (11), 3380-7. doi: 10.1158/1078-0432.CCR-06-2581.

Dutt, S., Narla, A., Lin, K., Mullally, A., Abayasekara, N., Megerdichian, C., Wilson, F. H., Currie, T., Khanna-Gupta, A., Berliner, N., Kutok, J. L. & Ebert, B. L. (2011). "Haploinsufficiency for ribosomal protein genes causes selective activation of p53 in human erythroid progenitor cells." *Blood*, *117* (9), 2567-76. doi: 10.1182/blood-2010-07-295238.

Ebert, B. L. (2009). "Deletion 5q in myelodysplastic syndrome: a paradigm for the study of hemizygous deletions in cancer." *Leukemia*, *23* (7), 1252-6. doi: 10.1038/leu.2009.53.

Ebert, B. L., Pretz, J., Bosco, J., Chang, C. Y., Tamayo, P., Galili, N., Raza, A., Root, D. E., Attar, E., Ellis, S. R. & Golub, T. R. (2008). "Identification of RPS14 as a 5q- syndrome gene by RNA interference screen." *Nature*, *451* (7176), 335-9. doi: 10.1038/nature06494.

Eisfeld, A. K., Marcucci, G., Maharry, K., Schwind, S., Radmacher, M. D., Nicolet, D., Becker, H., Mrozek, K., Whitman, S. P., Metzeler, K. H., Mendler, J. H., Wu, Y. Z., Liyanarachchi, S., Patel, R., Baer, M. R., Powell, B. L., Carter, T. H., Moore, J. O., Kolitz, J. E., Wetzler, M., Caligiuri, M. A., Larson, R. A., Tanner, S. M., de la Chapelle, A. & Bloomfield, C. D. (2012). "miR-3151 interplays with its host gene BAALC and independently affects outcome of patients with cytogenetically normal acute myeloid leukemia." *Blood*, *120* (2), 249-58. doi: 10.1182/blood-2012-02-408492.

Eisfeld, A. K., Schwind, S., Patel, R., Huang, X., Santhanam, R., Walker, C. J., Markowitz, J., Hoag, K. W., Jarvinen, T. M., Leffel, B., Perrotti, D., Carson, W. E., 3rd, Marcucci, G., Bloomfield, C. D. & de la Chapelle, A. (2014). "Intronic miR-3151 within BAALC drives leukemogenesis by deregulating the TP53 pathway." *Sci Signal*, *7* (321), ra36. doi: 10.1126/scisignal.2004762.

Elnenaei, M. O., Gruszka-Westwood, A. M., A'Hernt, R., Matutes, E., Sirohi, B., Powles, R. & Catovsky, D. (2003). "Gene abnormalities in multiple myeloma; the relevance of TP53, MDM2, and CDKN2A." *Haematologica*, *88* (5), 529-37.

Erba, H. P., Becker, P. S., Shami, P. J., Grunwald, M. R., Flesher, D. L., Zhu, M., Rasmussen, E., Henary, H. A., Anderson, A. A. & Wang, E. S. (2019). "Phase 1b study of the MDM2 inhibitor AMG 232 with or without trametinib in relapsed/refractory acute myeloid leukemia." *Blood Adv, 3* (13), 1939-1949. doi: 10.1182/ bloodadvances. 2019030916.

Eskelund, C. W., Dahl, C., Hansen, J. W., Westman, M., Kolstad, A., Pedersen, L. B., Montano-Almendras, C. P., Husby, S., Freiburghaus, C., Ek, S., Pedersen, A., Niemann, C., Raty, R., Brown, P., Geisler, C. H., Andersen, M. K., Guldberg, P., Jerkeman, M. & Gronbaek, K. (2017). "TP53 mutations identify younger mantle cell lymphoma patients who do not benefit from intensive chemoimmunotherapy." *Blood, 130* (17), 1903-1910. doi: 10.1182/blood-2017-04-779736.

Fabbri, G., Khiabanian, H., Holmes, A. B., Wang, J., Messina, M., Mullighan, C. G., Pasqualucci, L., Rabadan, R. & Dalla-Favera, R. (2013). "Genetic lesions associated with chronic lymphocytic leukemia transformation to Richter syndrome." *J Exp Med, 210* (11), 2273-88. doi: 10.1084/jem.20131448.

Faderl, S., Kantarjian, H. M., Estey, E., Manshouri, T., Chan, C. Y., Rahman Elsaied, A., Kornblau, S. M., Cortes, J., Thomas, D. A., Pierce, S., Keating, M. J., Estrov, Z. & Albitar, M. (2000). "The prognostic significance of p16(INK4a)/p14(ARF) locus deletion and MDM-2 protein expression in adult acute myelogenous leukemia." *Cancer, 89* (9), 1976-82. doi: 10.1002/1097-0142(20001101)89:9<1976::aid-cncr14>3.3.co;2-e.

Flynt, E., Bisht, K., Sridharan, V., Ortiz, M., Towfic, F. & Thakurta, A. (2020). "Prognosis, Biology, and Targeting of TP53 Dysregulation in Multiple Myeloma." *Cells, 9* (2). doi: 10.3390/cells9020287.

Fonseca, R., Blood, E., Rue, M., Harrington, D., Oken, M. M., Kyle, R. A., Dewald, G. W., Van Ness, B., Van Wier, S. A., Henderson, K. J., Bailey, R. J. & Greipp, P. R. (2003). "Clinical and biologic implications of recurrent genomic aberrations in myeloma." *Blood, 101* (11), 4569-75. doi: 10.1182/blood-2002-10-3017.

Fry, D. C., Wartchow, C., Graves, B., Janson, C., Lukacs, C., Kammlott, U., Belunis, C., Palme, S., Klein, C. & Vu, B. (2013). "Deconstruction of a nutlin: dissecting the binding determinants of a potent protein-protein interaction inhibitor." *ACS Med Chem Lett*, *4* (7), 660-5. doi: 10.1021/ml400062c.

Gaidano, G., Ballerini, P., Gong, J. Z., Inghirami, G., Neri, A., Newcomb, E. W., Magrath, I. T., Knowles, D. M. & Dalla-Favera, R. (1991). "p53 mutations in human lymphoid malignancies: association with Burkitt lymphoma and chronic lymphocytic leukemia." *Proc Natl Acad Sci U S A*, *88* (12), 5413-7. doi: 10.1073/pnas.88.12.5413.

Gao, L., Saeed, A., Golem, S., Zhang, D., Woodroof, J., McGuirk, J., Ganguly, S., Abhyankar, S., Lin, T. L. & Cui, W. (2020). "High-level MYC expression associates with poor survival in patients with acute myeloid leukemia and collaborates with overexpressed p53 in leukemic transformation in patients with myelodysplastic syndrome." *Int J Lab Hematol*. doi: 10.1111/ijlh.13316.

Gerbe, A., Alame, M., Dereure, O., Gonzalez, S., Durand, L., Tempier, A., De Oliveira, L., Tourneret, A., Costes-Martineau, V., Cacheux, V. & Szablewski, V. (2019). "Systemic, primary cutaneous, and breast implant-associated ALK-negative anaplastic large-cell lymphomas present similar biologic features despite distinct clinical behavior." *Virchows Arch*, *475* (2), 163-174. doi: 10.1007/s00428-019-02570-4.

Gluck, W. L., Gounder, M. M., Frank, R., Eskens, F., Blay, J. Y., Cassier, P. A., Soria, J. C., Chawla, S., de Weger, V., Wagner, A. J., Siegel, D., De Vos, F., Rasmussen, E. & Henary, H. A. (2020). "Phase 1 study of the MDM2 inhibitor AMG 232 in patients with advanced P53 wild-type solid tumors or multiple myeloma." *Invest New Drugs*, *38* (3), 831-843. doi: 10.1007/s10637-019-00840-1.

Greenberg, P. L., Tuechler, H., Schanz, J., Sanz, G., Garcia-Manero, G., Sole, F., Bennett, J. M., Bowen, D., Fenaux, P., Dreyfus, F., Kantarjian, H., Kuendgen, A., Levis, A., Malcovati, L., Cazzola, M., Cermak, J., Fonatsch, C., Le Beau, M. M., Slovak, M. L., Krieger, O., Luebbert, M., Maciejewski, J., Magalhaes, S. M., Miyazaki, Y., Pfeilstocker, M., Sekeres, M., Sperr, W. R., Stauder, R., Tauro, S., Valent, P., Vallespi,

T., van de Loosdrecht, A. A., Germing, U. & Haase, D. (2012). "Revised international prognostic scoring system for myelodysplastic syndromes." *Blood, 120* (12), 2454-65. doi: 10.1182/ blood-2012-03-420489.

Greiner, T. C., Moynihan, M. J., Chan, W. C., Lytle, D. M., Pedersen, A., Anderson, J. R. & Weisenburger, D. D. (1996). "p53 mutations in mantle cell lymphoma are associated with variant cytology and predict a poor prognosis." *Blood, 87* (10), 4302-10.

Gros, A., Laharanne, E., Vergier, M., Prochazkova-Carlotti, M., Pham-Ledard, A., Bandres, T., Poglio, S., Berhouet, S., Vergier, B., Vial, J. P., Chevret, E., Beylot-Barry, M. & Merlio, J. P. (2017). "TP53 alterations in primary and secondary Sezary syndrome: A diagnostic tool for the assessment of malignancy in patients with erythroderma." *PLoS One, 12* (3), e0173171. doi: 10.1371/journal.pone.0173171.

Gutierrez, N. C., Castellanos, M. V., Martin, M. L., Mateos, M. V., Hernandez, J. M., Fernandez, M., Carrera, D., Rosinol, L., Ribera, J. M., Ojanguren, J. M., Palomera, L., Gardella, S., Escoda, L., Hernandez-Boluda, J. C., Bello, J. L., de la Rubia, J., Lahuerta, J. J., San Miguel, J. F. & Gem Pethema Spanish Group. (2007). "Prognostic and biological implications of genetic abnormalities in multiple myeloma undergoing autologous stem cell transplantation: t(4;14) is the most relevant adverse prognostic factor, whereas RB deletion as a unique abnormality is not associated with adverse prognosis." *Leukemia, 21* (1), 143-50. doi: 10.1038/sj.leu.2404413.

Haase, D. (2008). "Cytogenetic features in myelodysplastic syndromes." *Ann Hematol, 87* (7), 515-26. doi: 10.1007/s00277-008-0483-y.

Haase, D., Stevenson, K. E., Neuberg, D., Maciejewski, J. P., Nazha, A., Sekeres, M. A., Ebert, B. L., Garcia-Manero, G., Haferlach, C., Haferlach, T., Kern, W., Ogawa, S., Nagata, Y., Yoshida, K., Graubert, T. A., Walter, M. J., List, A. F., Komrokji, R. S., Padron, E., Sallman, D., Papaemmanuil, E., Campbell, P. J., Savona, M. R., Seegmiller, A., Ades, L., Fenaux, P., Shih, L. Y., Bowen, D., Groves, M. J., Tauro, S., Fontenay, M., Kosmider, O., Bar-Natan, M., Steensma, D., Stone, R., Heuser, M., Thol, F., Cazzola, M., Malcovati, L., Karsan, A., Ganster,

C., Hellstrom-Lindberg, E., Boultwood, J., Pellagatti, A., Santini, V., Quek, L., Vyas, P., Tuchler, H., Greenberg, P. L., Bejar, R. & Molecular Prognostic Committee International Working Group for, M. D. S. (2019). "TP53 mutation status divides myelodysplastic syndromes with complex karyotypes into distinct prognostic subgroups." *Leukemia, 33* (7), 1747-1758. doi: 10.1038/s41375-018-0351-2.

Hafner, A., Bulyk, M. L., Jambhekar, A. & Lahav, G. (2019). "The multiple mechanisms that regulate p53 activity and cell fate." *Nat Rev Mol Cell Biol, 20* (4), 199-210. doi: 10.1038/s41580-019-0110-x.

Halldorsdottir, A. M., Lundin, A., Murray, F., Mansouri, L., Knuutila, S., Sundstrom, C., Laurell, A., Ehrencrona, H., Sander, B. & Rosenquist, R. (2011). "Impact of TP53 mutation and 17p deletion in mantle cell lymphoma." *Leukemia, 25* (12), 1904-8. doi: 10.1038/leu.2011.162.

Hallek, M. (2017). "Chronic lymphocytic leukemia: 2017 update on diagnosis, risk stratification, and treatment." *Am J Hematol, 92* (9), 946-965. doi: 10.1002/ajh.24826.

Han, X., Medeiros, L. J., Zhang, Y. H., You, M. J., Andreeff, M., Konopleva, M. & Bueso-Ramos, C. E. (2016). "High Expression of Human Homologue of Murine Double Minute 4 and the Short Splicing Variant, HDM4-S, in Bone Marrow in Patients With Acute Myeloid Leukemia or Myelodysplastic Syndrome." *Clin Lymphoma Myeloma Leuk, 16*, Suppl, S30-8. doi: 10.1016/j.clml.2016.03.012.

Handa, H., Murakami, Y., Ishihara, R., Kimura-Masuda, K. & Masuda, Y. (2019). "The Role and Function of microRNA in the Pathogenesis of Multiple Myeloma." *Cancers (Basel), 11* (11). doi: 10.3390/cancers11111738.

Hasegawa, H., Yamada, Y., Iha, H., Tsukasaki, K., Nagai, K., Atogami, S., Sugahara, K., Tsuruda, K., Ishizaki, A. & Kamihira, S. (2009). "Activation of p53 by Nutlin-3a, an antagonist of MDM2, induces apoptosis and cellular senescence in adult T-cell leukemia cells." *Leukemia, 23* (11), 2090-101. doi: 10.1038/leu.2009.171.

He, M., Gao, L., Zhang, S., Tao, L., Wang, J., Yang, J. & Zhu, M. (2014). "Prognostic significance of miR-34a and its target proteins of FOXP1, p53, and BCL2 in gastric MALT lymphoma and DLBCL." *Gastric Cancer*, *17* (3), 431-41. doi: 10.1007/s10120-013-0313-3.

Heavican, T. B., Bouska, A., Yu, J., Lone, W., Amador, C., Gong, Q., Zhang, W., Li, Y., Dave, B. J., Nairismagi, M. L., Greiner, T. C., Vose, J., Weisenburger, D. D., Lachel, C., Wang, C., Fu, K., Stevens, J. M., Lim, S. T., Ong, C. K., Gascoyne, R. D., Missiaglia, E., Lemonnier, F., Haioun, C., Hartmann, S., Pedersen, M. B., Laginestra, M. A., Wilcox, R. A., Teh, B. T., Yoshida, N., Ohshima, K., Seto, M., Rosenwald, A., Ott, G., Campo, E., Rimsza, L. M., Jaffe, E. S., Braziel, R. M., d'Amore, F., Inghirami, G., Bertoni, F., de Leval, L., Gaulard, P., Staudt, L. M., McKeithan, T. W., Pileri, S., Chan, W. C. & Iqbal, J. (2019). "Genetic drivers of oncogenic pathways in molecular subgroups of peripheral T-cell lymphoma." *Blood*, *133* (15), 1664-1676. doi: 10.1182/blood-2018-09-872549.

Her, N. G., Oh, J. W., Oh, Y. J., Han, S., Cho, H. J., Lee, Y., Ryu, G. H. & Nam, D. H. (2018). "Potent effect of the MDM2 inhibitor AMG232 on suppression of glioblastoma stem cells." *Cell Death Dis*, *9* (8), 792. doi: 10.1038/s41419-018-0825-1.

Hercher, C., Robain, M., Davi, F., Garand, R., Flandrin, G., Valensi, F., Vandeputte, H., Albert, A., Maynadie, M., Troussard, X., Simon, G. H., Lespinasse, J., Portefaix, G., Merle-Beral, H. * Cellulaire Groupe Francais d'Hematologie. (2001). "A multicentric study of 41 cases of B-prolymphocytic leukemia: two evolutive forms." *Leuk Lymphoma*, *42* (5), 981-7. doi: 10.3109/10428190109097717.

Hernandez, L., Fest, T., Cazorla, M., Teruya-Feldstein, J., Bosch, F., Peinado, M. A., Piris, M. A., Montserrat, E., Cardesa, A., Jaffe, E. S., Campo, E. & Raffeld, M. (1996). "p53 gene mutations and protein overexpression are associated with aggressive variants of mantle cell lymphomas." *Blood*, *87* (8), 3351-9.

Herrero, A. B., Rojas, E. A., Misiewicz-Krzeminska, I., Krzeminski, P. & Gutierrez, N. C. (2016). "Molecular Mechanisms of p53 Deregulation in Cancer: An Overview in Multiple Myeloma." *Int J Mol Sci*, *17* (12). doi: 10.3390/ijms17122003.

Hideshima, T., Mitsiades, C., Akiyama, M., Hayashi, T., Chauhan, D., Richardson, P., Schlossman, R., Podar, K., Munshi, N. C., Mitsiades, N. & Anderson, K. C. (2003). "Molecular mechanisms mediating antimyeloma activity of proteasome inhibitor PS-341." *Blood*, *101* (4), 1530-4. doi: 10.1182/blood-2002-08-2543.

Hof, J., Krentz, S., van Schewick, C., Korner, G., Shalapour, S., Rhein, P., Karawajew, L., Ludwig, W. D., Seeger, K., Henze, G., von Stackelberg, A., Hagemeier, C., Eckert, C. & Kirschner-Schwabe, R. (2011). "Mutations and deletions of the TP53 gene predict nonresponse to treatment and poor outcome in first relapse of childhood acute lymphoblastic leukemia." *J Clin Oncol*, *29* (23), 3185-93. doi: 10.1200/JCO.2011.34.8144.

Hunter, A. M. & Sallman, D. A. (2019). "Current status and new treatment approaches in TP53 mutated AML." *Best Pract Res Clin Haematol*, *32* (2), 134-144. doi: 10.1016/j.beha.2019.05.004.

Jadersten, M., Saft, L., Smith, A., Kulasekararaj, A., Pomplun, S., Gohring, G., Hedlund, A., Hast, R., Schlegelberger, B., Porwit, A., Hellstrom-Lindberg, E. & Mufti, G. J. (2011). "TP53 mutations in low-risk myelodysplastic syndromes with del(5q) predict disease progression." *J Clin Oncol*, *29* (15), 1971-9. doi: 10.1200/JCO.2010.31.8576.

Jaramillo Oquendo, C., Parker, H., Oscier, D., Ennis, S., Gibson, J. & Strefford, J. C. (2019). "Systematic Review of Somatic Mutations in Splenic Marginal Zone Lymphoma." *Sci Rep*, *9* (1), 10444. doi: 10.1038/s41598-019-46906-1.

Jaskova, Z., Pavlova, S., Malcikova, J., Brychtova, Y. & Trbusek, M. (2020). "PRIMA-1(MET) cytotoxic effect correlates with p53 protein reduction in TP53-mutated chronic lymphocytic leukemia cells." *Leuk Res*, *89*, 106288. doi: 10.1016/j.leukres.2019.106288.

Jin, L., Tabe, Y., Kojima, K., Zhou, Y., Pittaluga, S., Konopleva, M., Miida, T. & Raffeld, M. (2010). "MDM2 antagonist Nutlin-3 enhances bortezomib-mediated mitochondrial apoptosis in TP53-mutated mantle cell lymphoma." *Cancer Lett*, *299* (2), 161-70. doi: 10.1016/j.canlet.2010.08.015.

Jones, R. J., Bjorklund, C. C., Baladandayuthapani, V., Kuhn, D. J. & Orlowski, R. Z. (2012). "Drug resistance to inhibitors of the human double minute-2 E3 ligase is mediated by point mutations of p53, but can be overcome with the p53 targeting agent RITA." *Mol Cancer Ther*, *11* (10), 2243-53. doi: 10.1158/1535-7163.MCT-12-0135.

Kaindl, U., Morak, M., Portsmouth, C., Mecklenbrauker, A., Kauer, M., Zeginigg, M., Attarbaschi, A., Haas, O. A. & Panzer-Grumayer, R. (2014). "Blocking ETV6/RUNX1-induced MDM2 overexpression by Nutlin-3 reactivates p53 signaling in childhood leukemia." *Leukemia*, *28* (3), 600-8. doi: 10.1038/leu.2013.345.

Kang, M. H., Reynolds, C. P., Kolb, E. A., Gorlick, R., Carol, H., Lock, R., Keir, S. T., Maris, J. M., Wu, J., Lyalin, D., Kurmasheva, R. T., Houghton, P. J. & Smith, M. A. (2016). "Initial Testing (Stage 1) of MK-8242-A Novel MDM2 Inhibitor-by the Pediatric Preclinical Testing Program." *Pediatr Blood Cancer*, *63* (10), 1744-52. doi: 10.1002/pbc.26064.

Kawamura, M., Ohnishi, H., Guo, S. X., Sheng, X. M., Minegishi, M., Hanada, R., Horibe, K., Hongo, T., Kaneko, Y., Bessho, F., Yanagisawa, M., Sekiya, T. & Hayashi, Y. (1999). "Alterations of the p53, p21, p16, p15 and RAS genes in childhood T-cell acute lymphoblastic leukemia." *Leuk Res*, *23* (2), 115-26. doi: 10.1016/s0145-2126(98)00146-5.

Khurana, A. & Shafer, D. A. (2019). "MDM2 antagonists as a novel treatment option for acute myeloid leukemia: perspectives on the therapeutic potential of idasanutlin (RG7388)." *Onco Targets Ther*, *12*, 2903-2910. doi: 10.2147/OTT.S172315.

Kojima, K., Ishizawa, J. & Andreeff, M. (2016). "Pharmacological activation of wild-type p53 in the therapy of leukemia." *Exp Hematol*, *44* (9), 791-798. doi: 10.1016/j.exphem.2016.05.014.

Kojima, K., Konopleva, M., McQueen, T., O'Brien, S., Plunkett, W. & Andreeff, M. (2006). "Mdm2 inhibitor Nutlin-3a induces p53-mediated apoptosis by transcription-dependent and transcription-independent mechanisms and may overcome Atm-mediated resistance to fludarabine in chronic lymphocytic leukemia." *Blood*, *108* (3), 993-1000. doi: 10.1182/blood-2005-12-5148.

Kortum, K. M., Mai, E. K., Hanafiah, N. H., Shi, C. X., Zhu, Y. X., Bruins, L., Barrio, S., Jedlowski, P., Merz, M., Xu, J., Stewart, R. A., Andrulis, M., Jauch, A., Hillengass, J., Goldschmidt, H., Bergsagel, P. L., Braggio, E., Stewart, A. K. & Raab, M. S. (2016). "Targeted sequencing of refractory myeloma reveals a high incidence of mutations in CRBN and Ras pathway genes." *Blood*, *128* (9), 1226-33. doi: 10.1182/blood-2016-02-698092.

Krentz, S., Hof, J., Mendioroz, A., Vaggopoulou, R., Dorge, P., Lottaz, C., Engelmann, J. C., Groeneveld, T. W., Korner, G., Seeger, K., Hagemeier, C., Henze, G., Eckert, C., von Stackelberg, A. & Kirschner-Schwabe, R. (2013). "Prognostic value of genetic alterations in children with first bone marrow relapse of childhood B-cell precursor acute lymphoblastic leukemia." *Leukemia*, *27* (2), 295-304. doi: 10.1038/leu.2012.155.

Kridel, R., Chan, F. C., Mottok, A., Boyle, M., Farinha, P., Tan, K., Meissner, B., Bashashati, A., McPherson, A., Roth, A., Shumansky, K., Yap, D., Ben-Neriah, S., Rosner, J., Smith, M. A., Nielsen, C., Gine, E., Telenius, A., Ennishi, D., Mungall, A., Moore, R., Morin, R. D., Johnson, N. A., Sehn, L. H., Tousseyn, T., Dogan, A., Connors, J. M., Scott, D. W., Steidl, C., Marra, M. A., Gascoyne, R. D. & Shah, S. P. (2016). "Histological Transformation and Progression in Follicular Lymphoma: A Clonal Evolution Study." *PLoS Med*, *13* (12), e1002197. doi: 10.1371/journal.pmed.1002197.

Kulasekararaj, A. G., Smith, A. E., Mian, S. A., Mohamedali, A. M., Krishnamurthy, P., Lea, N. C., Gaken, J., Pennaneach, C., Ireland, R., Czepulkowski, B., Pomplun, S., Marsh, J. C. & Mufti, G. J. (2013). "TP53 mutations in myelodysplastic syndrome are strongly correlated with aberrations of chromosome 5, and correlate with adverse prognosis." *Br J Haematol*, *160* (5), 660-72. doi: 10.1111/bjh.12203.

Kumar, M., Lu, Z., Takwi, A. A., Chen, W., Callander, N. S., Ramos, K. S., Young, K. H. & Li, Y. (2011). "Negative regulation of the tumor suppressor p53 gene by microRNAs." *Oncogene*, *30* (7), 843-53. doi: 10.1038/onc.2010.457.

Lakshman, A., Painuly, U., Rajkumar, S. V., Ketterling, R. P., Kapoor, P., Greipp, P. T., Dispenzieri, A., Gertz, M. A., Buadi, F. K., Lacy, M. Q., Dingli, D., Fonder, A. L., Hayman, S. R., Hobbs, M. A., Gonsalves, W. I., Hwa, Y. L., Leung, N., Go, R. S., Lin, Y., Kourelis, T. V., Warsame, R., Lust, J. A., Russell, S. J., Zeldenrust, S. R., Kyle, R. A. & Kumar, S. K. (2019). "Impact of acquired del(17p) in multiple myeloma." *Blood Adv*, *3* (13), 1930-1938. doi: 10.1182/bloodadvances.2018028530.

Landau, D. A., Tausch, E., Taylor-Weiner, A. N., Stewart, C., Reiter, J. G., Bahlo, J., Kluth, S., Bozic, I., Lawrence, M., Bottcher, S., Carter, S. L., Cibulskis, K., Mertens, D., Sougnez, C. L., Rosenberg, M., Hess, J. M., Edelmann, J., Kless, S., Kneba, M., Ritgen, M., Fink, A., Fischer, K., Gabriel, S., Lander, E. S., Nowak, M. A., Dohner, H., Hallek, M., Neuberg, D., Getz, G., Stilgenbauer, S. & Wu, C. J. (2015). "Mutations driving CLL and their evolution in progression and relapse." *Nature*, *526* (7574), 525-30. doi: 10.1038/nature15395.

Lankenau, M. A., Patel, R., Liyanarachchi, S., Maharry, S. E., Hoag, K. W., Duggan, M., Walker, C. J., Markowitz, J., Carson, W. E., 3rd, Eisfeld, A. K. & de la Chapelle, A. (2015). "MicroRNA-3151 inactivates TP53 in BRAF-mutated human malignancies." *Proc Natl Acad Sci U S A* 112 (49):E6744-51. doi: 10.1073/pnas.1520390112.

Le, M. T., Teh, C., Shyh-Chang, N., Xie, H., Zhou, B., Korzh, V., Lodish, H. F. & Lim, B. (2009). "MicroRNA-125b is a novel negative regulator of p53." *Genes Dev*, *23* (7), 862-76. doi: 10.1101/gad.1767609.

Lee, J. H., List, A. & Sallman, D. A. (2019). "Molecular pathogenesis of myelodysplastic syndromes with deletion 5q." *Eur J Haematol*, *102* (3), 203-209. doi: 10.1111/ejh.13207.

Lehmann, S., Bykov, V. J. N., Ali, D., Andrén, O., Cherif, H., Tidefelt, U., Uggla, B., Yachnin, J., Juliusson, G., Moshfegh, A., Paul, C., Wiman, K. G. & Andersson, P. (2012). "Targeting p53 *in Vivo*: A First-In-Human Study With p53-targeting Compound APR-246 in Refractory Hematologic Malignancies and Prostate Cancer." *J Clin Oncol*, *30*(29), 3633-9. doi: 0.1200/JCO.2011.40.7783.

Leroy, K., Haioun, C., Lepage, E., Le Metayer, N., Berger, F., Labouyrie, E., Meignin, V., Petit, B., Bastard, C., Salles, G., Gisselbrecht, C.,

Reyes, F., Gaulard, P. & l'Adulte Groupe d'Etude des Lymphomes de. (2002). "p53 gene mutations are associated with poor survival in low and low-intermediate risk diffuse large B-cell lymphomas." *Ann Oncol*, *13* (7), 1108-15. doi: 10.1093/annonc/mdf185.

Leventaki, V., Rodic, V., Tripp, S. R., Bayerl, M. G., Perkins, S. L., Barnette, P., Schiffman, J. D. & Miles, R. R. (2012). "TP53 pathway analysis in paediatric Burkitt lymphoma reveals increased MDM4 expression as the only TP53 pathway abnormality detected in a subset of cases." *Br J Haematol*, *158* (6), 763-71. doi: 10.1111/j.1365-2141.2012.09243.x.

Li, L., Tan, Y., Chen, X., Xu, Z., Yang, S., Ren, F., Guo, H., Wang, X., Chen, Y., Li, G. & Wang, H. (2014). "MDM4 overexpressed in acute myeloid leukemia patients with complex karyotype and wild-type TP53." *PLoS One*, *9* (11), e113088. doi: 10.1371/journal.pone.0113088.

Linggi, B., Muller-Tidow, C., van de Locht, L., Hu, M., Nip, J., Serve, H., Berdel, W. E., van der Reijden, B., Quelle, D. E., Rowley, J. D., Cleveland, J., Jansen, J. H., Pandolfi, P. P. & Hiebert, S. W. (2002). "The t(8;21) fusion protein, AML1 ETO, specifically represses the transcription of the p14(ARF) tumor suppressor in acute myeloid leukemia." *Nat Med*, *8* (7), 743-50. doi: 10.1038/nm726.

Lionetti, M., Agnelli, L., Mosca, L., Fabris, S., Andronache, A., Todoerti, K., Ronchetti, D., Deliliers, G. L. & Neri, A. (2009). "Integrative high-resolution microarray analysis of human myeloma cell lines reveals deregulated miRNA expression associated with allelic imbalances and gene expression profiles." *Genes Chromosomes Cancer*, *48* (6), 521-31. doi: 10.1002/gcc.20660.

Lionetti, M., Biasiolo, M., Agnelli, L., Todoerti, K., Mosca, L., Fabris, S., Sales, G., Deliliers, G. L., Bicciato, S., Lombardi, L., et al. (2009). "Identification of microRNA expression patterns and definition of a microRNA/mRNA regulatory network in distinct molecular groups of multiple myeloma." *Blood*, *114*, e20–e26.

Lode, L., Eveillard, M., Trichet, V., Soussi, T., Wuilleme, S., Richebourg, S., Magrangeas, F., Ifrah, N., Campion, L., Traulle, C., Guilhot, F.,

Caillot, D., Marit, G., Mathiot, C., Facon, T., Attal, M., Harousseau, J. L., Moreau, P., Minvielle, S. & Avet-Loiseau, H. (2010). "Mutations in TP53 are exclusively associated with del(17p) in multiple myeloma." *Haematologica, 95* (11), 1973-6. doi: 10.3324/ haematol.2010.023697.

Loghavi, S., Al-Ibraheemi, A., Zuo, Z., Garcia-Manero, G., Yabe, M., Wang, S. A., Kantarjian, H. M., Yin, C. C., Miranda, R. N., Luthra, R., Medeiros, L. J., Bueso-Ramos, C. E. & Khoury, J. D. (2015). "TP53 overexpression is an independent adverse prognostic factor in de novo myelodysplastic syndromes with fibrosis." *Br J Haematol, 171* (1), 91-9. doi: 10.1111/bjh.13529.

Lopez-Anglada, L., Gutierrez, N. C., Garcia, J. L., Mateos, M. V., Flores, T. & San Miguel, J. F. (2010). "P53 deletion may drive the clinical evolution and treatment response in multiple myeloma." *Eur J Haematol, 84* (4), 359-61. doi: 10.1111/j.1600-0609.2009.01399.x.

Love, C., Sun, Z., Jima, D., Li, G., Zhang, J., Miles, R., Richards, K. L., Dunphy, C. H., Choi, W. W., Srivastava, G., Lugar, P. L., Rizzieri, D. A., Lagoo, A. S., Bernal-Mizrachi, L., Mann, K. P., Flowers, C. R., Naresh, K. N., Evens, A. M., Chadburn, A., Gordon, L. I., Czader, M. B., Gill, J. I., Hsi, E. D., Greenough, A., Moffitt, A. B., McKinney, M., Banerjee, A., Grubor, V., Levy, S., Dunson, D. B. & Dave, S. S. (2012). "The genetic landscape of mutations in Burkitt lymphoma." *Nat Genet, 44* (12), 1321-5. doi: 10.1038/ng.2468.

Lu, T. X., Young, K. H., Xu, W. & Li, J. Y. (2016). "TP53 dysfunction in diffuse large B-cell lymphoma." *Crit Rev Oncol Hematol, 97*, 47-55. doi: 10.1016/j.critrevonc.2015.08.006.

Lundberg, P., Karow, A., Nienhold, R., Looser, R., Hao-Shen, H., Nissen, I., Girsberger, S., Lehmann, T., Passweg, J., Stern, M., Beisel, C., Kralovics, R. & Skoda, R. C. (2014). "Clonal evolution and clinical correlates of somatic mutations in myeloproliferative neoplasms." *Blood, 123* (14), 2220-8. doi: 10.1182/blood-2013-11-537167.

Luo, Q., Pan, W., Zhou, S., Wang, G., Yi, H., Yang, L., Yan, X., Yuan, L., Wang, J., Liu, Z., Chen, H., Qiu, M., Yang, D. & Sun, J. (2020). "A novel BCL-2 inhibitor APG-2575 exerts synthetic lethality with BTK or

MDM2-P53 inhibitor in Diffuse Large B-Cell Lymphoma." *Oncol Res.* doi: 10.3727/096504020X15825405463920.

Luo, Z., Cui, R., Tili, E. & Croce, C. (2018). "Friend or Foe: MicroRNAs in the p53 network." *Cancer Lett*, *419*, 96-102. doi: 10.1016/j.canlet.2018.01.013.

Manfe, V., Biskup, E., Johansen, P., Kamstrup, M. R., Krejsgaard, T. F., Morling, N., Wulf, H. C. & Gniadecki, R. (2012). "MDM2 inhibitor nutlin-3a induces apoptosis and senescence in cutaneous T-cell lymphoma: role of p53." *J Invest Dermatol*, *132* (5), 1487-96. doi: 10.1038/jid.2012.10.

Marisavljevic, D., Rolovic, Z., Panitic, M., Novak, A., Djordjevic, V., Lazarevic, V., Boskovic, D. & Colovic, M. (2004). "[Chromosome 17 abnormalities in patients with primary myelodysplastic syndrome: incidence and biologic significance]." *Srp Arh Celok Lek*, *132* (1-2), 10-3. doi: 10.2298/sarh0402010m.

Maslah, N., Salomao, N., Drevon, L., Verger, E., Partouche, N., Ly, P., Aubin, P., Naoui, N., Schlageter, M. H., Bally, C., Miekoutima, E., Rahme, R., Lehmann-Che, J., Ades, L., Fenaux, P., Cassinat, B. & Giraudier, S. (2019). "Synergistic effects of PRIMA-1Met (APR-246) and Azacitidine in TP53-mutated myelodysplastic syndromes and acute myeloid leukemia." *Haematologica*. doi: 10.3324/ haematol.2019.218453.

McGraw, K. L., Nguyen, J., Komrokji, R. S., Sallman, D., Al Ali, N. H., Padron, E., Lancet, J. E., Moscinski, L. C., List, A. F. & Zhang, L. (2016). "Immunohistochemical pattern of p53 is a measure of TP53 mutation burden and adverse clinical outcome in myelodysplastic syndromes and secondary acute myeloid leukemia." *Haematologica*, *101* (8), e320-3. doi: 10.3324/haematol.2016.143214.

Merz, M., Hielscher, T., Seckinger, A., Hose, D., Mai, E. K., Raab, M. S., Goldschmidt, H., Jauch, A. & Hillengass, J. (2016). "Baseline characteristics, chromosomal alterations, and treatment affecting prognosis of deletion 17p in newly diagnosed myeloma." *Am J Hematol*, *91* (11), E473-E477. doi: 10.1002/ajh.24533.

Misiewicz-Krzeminska, I., Krzeminski, P., Corchete, L. A., Quwaider, D., Rojas, E. A., Herrero, A. B. & Gutierrez, N. C. (2019). "Factors Regulating microRNA Expression and Function in Multiple Myeloma." *Noncoding RNA*, *5* (1). doi: 10.3390/ncrna5010009.

Moll, U. & Petrenko, O. (2003). "The MDM2-p53 interaction." *Mol Cancer Res.*, *1*(14), 1001-1008.

Molteni, A., Ravano, E., Riva, M., Nichelatti, M., Bandiera, L., Crucitti, L., Truini, M. & Cairoli, R. (2019). "Prognostic Impact of Immunohistochemical p53 Expression in Bone Marrow Biopsy in Higher Risk MDS: a Pilot Study." *Mediterr J Hematol Infect Dis*, *11* (1), e2019015. doi: 10.4084/MJHID.2019.015.

Montalban-Bravo, G., Kanagal-Shamanna, R., Benton, C. B., Class, C. A., Chien, K. S., Sasaki, K., Naqvi, K., Alvarado, Y., Kadia, T. M., Ravandi, F., Daver, N., Takahashi, K., Jabbour, E., Borthakur, G., Pemmaraju, N., Konopleva, M., Soltysiak, K. A., Pierce, S. R., Bueso-Ramos, C. E., Patel, K. P., Kantarjian, H. & Garcia-Manero, G. (2020). "Genomic context and TP53 allele frequency define clinical outcomes in TP53-mutated myelodysplastic syndromes." *Blood Adv*, *4* (3), 482-495. doi: 10.1182/bloodadvances.2019001101.

Monti, S., Chapuy, B., Takeyama, K., Rodig, S. J., Hao, Y., Yeda, K. T., Inguilizian, H., Mermel, C., Currie, T., Dogan, A., Kutok, J. L., Beroukhim, R., Neuberg, D., Habermann, T. M., Getz, G., Kung, A. L., Golub, T. R. & Shipp, M. A. (2012). "Integrative analysis reveals an outcome-associated and targetable pattern of p53 and cell cycle deregulation in diffuse large B cell lymphoma." *Cancer Cell*, *22* (3), 359-72. doi: 10.1016/j.ccr.2012.07.014.

Morgan, G. J., Walker, B. A. & Davies, F. E. (2012). "The genetic architecture of multiple myeloma." *Nat Rev Cancer*, *12* (5), 335-48. doi: 10.1038/nrc3257.

Muller-Tidow, C., Metzelder, S. K., Buerger, H., Packeisen, J., Ganser, A., Heil, G., Kugler, K., Adiguzel, G., Schwable, J., Steffen, B., Ludwig, W. D., Heinecke, A., Buchner, T., Berdel, W. E. & Serve, H. (2004). "Expression of the p14ARF tumor suppressor predicts survival in acute myeloid leukemia." *Leukemia*, *18* (4), 720-6. doi: 10.1038/sj.leu.2403296.

Nabhan, C. & Rosen, S. T. (2014). "Chronic lymphocytic leukemia: a clinical review." *JAMA*, *312* (21), 2265-76. doi: 10.1001/jama.2014.14553.

Nahi, H., Lehmann, S., Mollgard, L., Bengtzen, S., Selivanova, G., Wiman, K. G., Paul, C. & Merup, M. (2004). "Effects of PRIMA-1 on chronic lymphocytic leukaemia cells with and without hemizygous p53 deletion." *Br J Haematol*, *127* (3), 285-91. doi: 10.1111/j.1365-2141.2004.05210.x.

Nahi, H., Merup, M., Lehmann, S., Bengtzen, S., Mollgard, L., Selivanova, G., Wiman, K. G. & Paul, C. (2006). "PRIMA-1 induces apoptosis in acute myeloid leukaemia cells with p53 gene deletion." *Br J Haematol*, *132* (2), 230-6. doi: 10.1111/j.1365-2141.2005.05851.x.

Namiki, T., Sakashita, A., Kobayashi, H., Maseki, N., Izumo, T., Komada, Y., Koizumi, S., Shikano, T., Kikuta, A., Watanabe, A., Suzumiya, J., Kikuchi, M. & Kaneko, Y. (2003). "Clinical and genetic characteristics of Japanese Burkitt lymphomas with or without leukemic presentation." *Int J Hematol*, *77* (5), 490-8. doi: 10.1007/ BF02986618.

Nishiwaki, S., Ito, M., Watarai, R., Okuno, S., Harada, Y., Yamamoto, S., Suzuki, K., Kurahashi, S., Iwasaki, T. & Sugiura, I. (2016). "A new prognostic index to make short-term prognoses in MDS patients treated with azacitidine: A combination of p53 expression and cytogenetics." *Leuk Res*, *41*, 21-6. doi: 10.1016/j.leukres.2015.11.014.

O'Shea, D., O'Riain, C., Taylor, C., Waters, R., Carlotti, E., Macdougall, F., Gribben, J., Rosenwald, A., Ott, G., Rimsza, L. M., Smeland, E. B., Johnson, N., Campo, E., Greiner, T. C., Chan, W. C., Gascoyne, R. D., Wright, G., Staudt, L. M., Lister, T. A. & Fitzgibbon, J. (2008). "The presence of TP53 mutation at diagnosis of follicular lymphoma identifies a high-risk group of patients with shortened time to disease progression and poorer overall survival." *Blood*, *112* (8), 3126-9. doi: 10.1182/blood-2008-05-154013.

Ok, C. Y., Patel, K. P., Garcia-Manero, G., Routbort, M. J., Peng, J., Tang, G., Goswami, M., Young, K. H., Singh, R., Medeiros, L. J., Kantarjian,

H. M., Luthra, R. & Wang, S. A. (2015). "TP53 mutation characteristics in therapy-related myelodysplastic syndromes and acute myeloid leukemia is similar to de novo diseases." *J Hematol Oncol*, *8*, 45. doi: 10.1186/s13045-015-0139-z.

Onaindia, A., Medeiros, L. J. & Patel, K. P. (2017). "Clinical utility of recently identified diagnostic, prognostic, and predictive molecular biomarkers in mature B-cell neoplasms." *Mod Pathol*, *30* (10), 1338-1366. doi: 10.1038/modpathol.2017.58.

Parry, M., Rose-Zerilli, M. J., Ljungstrom, V., Gibson, J., Wang, J., Walewska, R., Parker, H., Parker, A., Davis, Z., Gardiner, A., McIver-Brown, N., Kalpadakis, C., Xochelli, A., Anagnostopoulos, A., Fazi, C., de Castro, D. G., Dearden, C., Pratt, G., Rosenquist, R., Ashton-Key, M., Forconi, F., Collins, A., Ghia, P., Matutes, E., Pangalis, G., Stamatopoulos, K., Oscier, D. & Strefford, J. C. (2015). "Genetics and Prognostication in Splenic Marginal Zone Lymphoma: Revelations from Deep Sequencing." *Clin Cancer Res*, *21* (18), 4174-4183. doi: 10.1158/1078-0432.CCR-14-2759.

Pasqualucci, L., Khiabanian, H., Fangazio, M., Vasishtha, M., Messina, M., Holmes, A. B., Ouillette, P., Trifonov, V., Rossi, D., Tabbo, F., Ponzoni, M., Chadburn, A., Murty, V. V., Bhagat, G., Gaidano, G., Inghirami, G., Malek, S. N., Rabadan, R. & Dalla-Favera, R. (2014). "Genetics of follicular lymphoma transformation." *Cell Rep*, *6* (1), 130-40. doi: 10.1016/j.celrep.2013.12.027.

Paul, T. A., Bies, J., Small, D. & Wolff, L. (2010). "Signatures of polycomb repression and reduced H3K4 trimethylation are associated with p15INK4b DNA methylation in AML." *Blood*, *115* (15), 3098-108. doi: 10.1182/blood-2009-07-233858.

Peller, S. & Rotter, V. (2003). "TP53 in hematological cancer: low incidence of mutations with significant clinical relevance." *Hum Mutat*, *21* (3), 277-84. doi: 10.1002/humu.10190.

Pichiorri, F., Suh, S. S., Ladetto, M., Kuehl, M., Palumbo, T., Drandi, D., Taccioli, C., Zanesi, N., Alder, H., Hagan, J. P., Munker, R., Volinia, S., Boccadoro, M., Garzon, R., Palumbo, A., Aqeilan, R. I. & Croce, C. M. (2008). "MicroRNAs regulate critical genes associated with multiple myeloma pathogenesis." *Proc Natl Acad Sci U S A*, *105* (35), 12885-90. doi: 10.1073/pnas.0806202105.

Pichiorri, F., Suh, S. S., Rocci, A., De Luca, L., Taccioli, C., Santhanam, R., Zhou, W., Benson, D. M., Jr. Hofmainster, C., Alder, H., Garofalo, M., Di Leva, G., Volinia, S., Lin, H. J., Perrotti, D., Kuehl, M., Aqeilan, R. I., Palumbo, A. & Croce, C. M. (2010). "Downregulation of p53-inducible microRNAs 192, 194, and 215 impairs the p53/MDM2 autoregulatory loop in multiple myeloma development." *Cancer Cell*, *18* (4), 367-81. doi: 10.1016/j.ccr.2010.09.005.

Piris, M. A., Onaindia, A. & Mollejo, M. (2017). "Splenic marginal zone lymphoma." *Best Pract Res Clin Haematol*, *30* (1-2), 56-64. doi: 10.1016/j.beha.2016.09.005.

Preudhomme, C., Dervite, I., Wattel, E., Vanrumbeke, M., Flactif, M., Lai, J. L., Hecquet, B., Coppin, M. C., Nelken, B., Gosselin, B., et al. (1995). "Clinical significance of p53 mutations in newly diagnosed Burkitt's lymphoma and acute lymphoblastic leukemia: a report of 48 cases." *J Clin Oncol*, *13* (4), 812-20. doi: 10.1200/JCO.1995.13.4.812.

Prokocimer, M., Molchadsky, A. & Rotter, V. (2017). "Dysfunctional diversity of p53 proteins in adult acute myeloid leukemia: projections on diagnostic workup and therapy." *Blood*, *130* (6), 699-712. doi: 10.1182/blood-2017-02-763086.

Qi, S. M., Cheng, G., Cheng, X. D., Xu, Z., Xu, B., Zhang, W. D. & Qin. J. J. (2020). "Targeting USP7-Mediated Deubiquitination of MDM2/MDMX-p53 Pathway for Cancer Therapy: Are We There Yet?" *Front Cell Dev Biol*, *8*, 233. doi: 10.3389/fcell.2020.00233.

Qu, X., Li, H., Braziel, R. M., Passerini, V., Rimsza, L. M., Hsi, E. D., Leonard, J. P., Smith, S. M., Kridel, R., Press, O., Weigert, O., LeBlanc, M., Friedberg, J. W. & Fang, M. (2019). "Genomic alterations important for the prognosis in patients with follicular lymphoma treated in SWOG study S0016." *Blood*, *133* (1), 81-93. doi: 10.1182/blood-2018-07-865428.

Quesnel, B., Preudhomme, C., Oscier, D., Lepelley, P., Collyn-d'Hooghe, M., Facon, T., Zandecki, M. & Fenaux, P. (1994). "Over-expression of the MDM2 gene is found in some cases of haematological malignancies." *Br J Haematol,* 88 (2), 415-8. doi: 10.1111/j.1365-2141.1994.tb05044.x.

Quintás-Cardama, A., Hu, C., Qutub, A., Qiu, Y. H., Zhang, X., Post, S. M., Zhang, N., Coombes, K. & Kornblau, S. M. (2017). "p53 Pathway Dysfunction Is Highly Prevalent in Acute Myeloid Leukemia Independent of TP53 Mutational Status." *Leukemia,* 31(6), 1296-1305. doi: DOI: 10.1038/leu.2016.350.

Rajkumar, S. V. (2016). "Multiple myeloma: 2016 update on diagnosis, risk-stratification, and management." *Am J Hematol,* 91 (7), 719-34. doi: 10.1002/ajh.24402.

Ramos, F., Robledo, C., Izquierdo-Garcia, F. M., Suarez-Vilela, D., Benito, R., Fuertes, M., Insunza, A., Barragan, E., Del Rey, M., Garcia-Ruiz de Morales, J. M., Tormo, M., Salido, E., Zamora, L., Pedro, C., Sanchez-Del-Real, J., Diez-Campelo, M., Del Canizo, C., Sanz, G. F., Hernandez-Rivas, J. M. & Syndromes Spanish Group for Myelodysplastic. (2016). "Bone marrow fibrosis in myelodysplastic syndromes: a prospective evaluation including mutational analysis." *Oncotarget,* 7 (21), 30492-503. doi: 10.18632/oncotarget.9026.

Rampal, R., Ahn, J., Abdel-Wahab, O., Nahas, M., Wang, K., Lipson, D., Otto, G. A., Yelensky, R., Hricik, T., McKenney, A. S., Chiosis, G., Chung, Y. R., Pandey, S., van den Brink, M. R., Armstrong, S. A., Dogan, A., Intlekofer, A., Manshouri, T., Park, C. Y., Verstovsek, S., Rapaport, F., Stephens, P. J., Miller, V. A. & Levine, R. L. (2014). "Genomic and functional analysis of leukemic transformation of myeloproliferative neoplasms." *Proc Natl Acad Sci U S A,* 111 (50), E5401-10. doi: 10.1073/pnas.1407792111.

Rassidakis, G. Z., Thomaides, A., Wang, S., Jiang, Y., Fourtouna, A., Lai, R. & Medeiros, L. J. (2005). "p53 gene mutations are uncommon but p53 is commonly expressed in anaplastic large-cell lymphoma." *Leukemia,* 19 (9),1663-9. doi: 10.1038/sj.leu.2403840.

Ravandi, F., Gojo, I., Patnaik, M. M., Minden, M. D., Kantarjian, H., Johnson-Levonas, A. O., Fancourt, C., Lam, R., Jones, M. B., Knox, C. D., Rose, S., Patel, P. S. & Tibes, R. (2016). "A phase I trial of the human double minute 2 inhibitor (MK-8242) in patients with refractory/recurrent acute myelogenous leukemia (AML)." *Leuk Res*, *48*, 92-100. doi: 10.1016/j.leukres.2016.07.004.

Reece, D., Song, K. W., Fu, T., Roland, B., Chang, H., Horsman, D. E., Mansoor, A., Chen, C., Masih-Khan, E., Trieu, Y., Bruyere, H., Stewart, D. A. & Bahlis, N. J. (2009). "Influence of cytogenetics in patients with relapsed or refractory multiple myeloma treated with lenalidomide plus dexamethasone: adverse effect of deletion 17p13." *Blood, 114* (3), 522-5. doi: 10.1182/blood-2008-12-193458.

Richardson, A. I., Yin, C. C., Cui, W., Li, N., Medeiros, L. J., Li, L. & Zhang, D. (2019). "p53 and beta-Catenin Expression Predict Poorer Prognosis in Patients With Anaplastic Large-Cell Lymphoma." *Clin Lymphoma Myeloma Leuk, 19* (7), e385-e392. doi: 10.1016/j.clml.2019.03.030.

Richardson, A. I., Zhang, D., Woodroof, J. & Cui, W. (2019). "p53 expression in large B-cell lymphomas with MYC extra copies and CD99 expression in large B-cell lymphomas in relation to MYC status." *Hum Pathol, 86*, 21-31. doi: 10.1016/j.humpath.2018.11.015.

Richmond, J., Carol, H., Evans, K., et al. (2015). "Effective targeting of the P53-MDM2 axis in preclinical models of infant MLL-rearranged acute lymphoblastic leukemia." *EClin Cancer Res., 21*(6), 1395- 1405. doi: https://doi.org/10.1158/1078-0432.CCR-14-2300.

Rossi, D., Cerri, M., Deambrogi, C., Sozzi, E., Cresta, S., Rasi, S., De Paoli, L., Spina, V., Gattei, V., Capello, D., Forconi, F., Lauria, F. & Gaidano, G. (2009). "The prognostic value of TP53 mutations in chronic lymphocytic leukemia is independent of Del17p13: implications for overall survival and chemorefractoriness." *Clin Cancer Res, 15* (3), 995-1004. doi: 10.1158/1078-0432.CCR-08-1630.

Rossi, D., Spina, V., Deambrogi, C., Rasi, S., Laurenti, L., Stamatopoulos, K., Arcaini, L., Lucioni, M., Rocque, G. B., Xu-Monette, Z. Y., Visco, C., Chang, J., Chigrinova, E., Forconi, F., Marasca, R., Besson, C., Papadaki, T., Paulli, M., Larocca, L. M., Pileri, S. A., Gattei, V., Bertoni, F., Foa, R., Young, K. H. & Gaidano, G. (2011). "The genetics of Richter syndrome reveals disease heterogeneity and predicts survival after transformation." *Blood, 117* (12), 3391-401. doi: 10.1182/blood-2010-09-302174.

Rucker, F. G., Russ, A. C., Cocciardi, S., Kett, H., Schlenk, R. F., Botzenhardt, U., Langer, C., Krauter, J., Frohling, S., Schlegelberger, B., Ganser, A., Lichter, P., Zenz, T., Dohner, H., Dohner, K. & Bullinger, L. (2013). "Altered miRNA and gene expression in acute myeloid leukemia with complex karyotype identify networks of prognostic relevance." *Leukemia, 27* (2), 353-61. doi: 10.1038/leu.2012.208.

Saft, L., Karimi, M., Ghaderi, M., Matolcsy, A., Mufti, G. J., Kulasekararaj, A., Gohring, G., Giagounidis, A., Selleslag, D., Muus, P., Sanz, G., Mittelman, M., Bowen, D., Porwit, A., Fu, T., Backstrom, J., Fenaux, P., MacBeth, K. J. & Hellstrom-Lindberg, E. (2014). "p53 protein expression independently predicts outcome in patients with lower-risk myelodysplastic syndromes with del(5q)." *Haematologica, 99* (6), 1041-9. doi: 10.3324/haematol.2013.098103.

Saha, M. N., Chen, Y., Chen, M. H., Chen, G. & Chang, H. (2014). "Small molecule MIRA-1 induces *in vitro* and *in vivo* anti-myeloma activity and synergizes with current anti-myeloma agents." *Br J Cancer, 110* (9), 2224-31. doi: 10.1038/bjc.2014.164.

Saha, M. N., Jiang, H. & Chang, H. (2010). "Molecular mechanisms of nutlin-induced apoptosis in multiple myeloma: evidence for p53-transcription-dependent and -independent pathways." *Cancer Biol Ther, 10* (6), 567-78. doi: 10.4161/cbt.10.6.12535.

Saha, M. N., Jiang, H., Jayakar, J., Reece, D., Branch, D. R. & Chang, H. (2010). "MDM2 antagonist nutlin plus proteasome inhibitor velcade combination displays a synergistic anti-myeloma activity." *Cancer Biol Ther, 9* (11), 936-44. doi: 10.4161/cbt.9.11.11882.

Saha, M. N., Jiang, H., Mukai, A. & Chang, H. (2010). "RITA inhibits multiple myeloma cell growth through induction of p53-mediated caspase-dependent apoptosis and synergistically enhances nutlin-induced cytotoxic responses." *Mol Cancer Ther, 9* (11), 3041-51. doi: 10.1158/1535-7163.MCT-10-0471.

Saha, M. N., Jiang, H., Yang, Y., Reece, D. & Chang, H. (2013). "PRIMA-1Met/APR-246 displays high antitumor activity in multiple myeloma by induction of p73 and Noxa." *Mol Cancer Ther*, *12* (11), 2331-41. doi: 10.1158/1535-7163.MCT-12-1166.

Saha, M. N., Jiang, H., Yang, Y., Zhu, X., Wang, X., Schimmer, A. D., Qiu, L. & Chang, H. (2012). "Targeting p53 via JNK pathway: a novel role of RITA for apoptotic signaling in multiple myeloma." *PLoS One*, *7* (1), e30215. doi: 10.1371/journal.pone.0030215.

Saha, M. N., Qiu, L. & Chang, H. (2013). "Targeting p53 by small molecules in hematological malignancies." *J Hematol Oncol*, *6*, 23. doi: 10.1186/1756-8722-6-23.

Sakhdari, A., Ok, C. Y., Patel, K. P., Kanagal-Shamanna, R., Yin, C. C., Zuo, Z., Hu, S., Routbort, M. J., Luthra, R., Medeiros, L. J., Khoury, J. D. & Loghavi, S. (2019). "TP53 mutations are common in mantle cell lymphoma, including the indolent leukemic non-nodal variant." *Ann Diagn Pathol*, *41*, 38-42. doi: 10.1016/j.anndiagpath.2019.05.004.

Salido, M., Baro, C., Oscier, D., Stamatopoulos, K., Dierlamm, J., Matutes, E., Traverse-Glehen, A., Berger, F., Felman, P., Thieblemont, C., Gesk, S., Athanasiadou, A., Davis, Z., Gardiner, A., Milla, F., Ferrer, A., Mollejo, M., Calasanz, M. J., Florensa, L., Espinet, B., Luno, E., Wlodarska, I., Verhoef, G., Garcia-Granero, M., Salar, A., Papadaki, T., Serrano, S., Piris, M. A. & Sole, F. (2010). "Cytogenetic aberrations and their prognostic value in a series of 330 splenic marginal zone B-cell lymphomas: a multicenter study of the Splenic B-Cell Lymphoma Group." *Blood*, *116* (9), 1479-88. doi: 10.1182/blood-2010-02-267476.

Sallman, D. A., Komrokji, R., Vaupel, C., Cluzeau, T., Geyer, S. M., McGraw, K. L., Al Ali, N. H., Lancet, J., McGinniss, M. J., Nahas, S., Smith, A. E., Kulasekararaj, A., Mufti, G., List, A., Hall, J. & Padron, E. (2016). "Impact of TP53 mutation variant allele frequency on phenotype and outcomes in myelodysplastic syndromes." *Leukemia*, *30* (3), 666-73. doi: 10.1038/leu.2015.304.

Sallman, D. A., Borate, U., Cull, E. H., Donnellan, W. B., Komrokji, R. S., Steidl, U. G., Corvez, M. M., Payton, M., Annis, D. A., Pinchasik, D., Aivado, M. & Verma, A (2018). "Phase 1/1b Study of the Stapled

Peptide ALRN-6924, a Dual Inhibitor of MDMX and MDM2, As Monotherapy or in Combination with Cytarabine for the Treatment of Relapsed/Refractory AML and Advanced MDS with TP53 Wild-Type D." *Blood*, *132*, (Supplement 1), 4066. doi: https://doi.org/ 10.1182/blood-2018-99-118780.

Sallman, D. A., DeZern, A. E., Steensma, D. P., Sweet, K. L., Cluzeau, T., Sekeres, M. A., Garcia-Manero, G., Roboz, G. J., McLemore, A. F., McGraw, K. L., Puskas, J., Zhang, L., Bhagat, C. K., Yao, J., Al Ali, N., Padron, E., Tell, R., Lancet, J. E., Fenaux, P., List, A. F. & Komrokji, R. S. (2018). "Phase 1b/2 Combination Study of APR-246 and Azacitidine (AZA) in Patients with TP53 mutant Myelodysplastic Syndromes (MDS) and Acute Myeloid Leukemia (AML)." *Blood*, *132*, doi: https://doi.org/10.1182/blood-2018-99-119990.

Sallman, D. A., DeZern, A. E., Garcia-Manero, G., Steensma, D. P., Roboz, G. J., Sekeres, M. A., Cluzeau, T., Sweet, K. L., McLemore, A. F., McGraw, K.., Puskas, J.., Zhang, L., Yao, J., Mo, Q., Nardelli, L., Al Ali, N., Padron, E., Korbel, G., Attar, E. C., Kantarjian, H. M., Lancet, J. E., Fenaux, P., List, A. F. & Komrokji, R. S. (2019). "Phase 2 Results of APR-246 and Azacitidine (AZA) in Patients with TP53 mutant Myelodysplastic Syndromes (MDS) and Oligoblastic Acute Myeloid Leukemia (AML)." *Blood*, *134*, (Supplement_1), 676, 134.

Salmoiraghi, S., Rambaldi, A. & Spinelli, O. (2018). "TP53 in adult acute lymphoblastic leukemia." *Leuk Lymphoma*, *59* (4), 778-789. doi: 10.1080/10428194.2017.1344839.

Schieber, M., Gordon, L. I. & Karmali, R. (2018). "Current overview and treatment of mantle cell lymphoma." *F1000Res*, *7*. doi: 10.12688/f1000research.14122.1.

Schneider, R. K., Schenone, M., Ferreira, M. V., Kramann, R., Joyce, C. E., Hartigan, C., Beier, F., Brummendorf, T. H., Germing, U., Platzbecker, U., Busche, G., Knuchel, R., Chen, M. C., Waters, C. S., Chen, E., Chu, L. P., Novina, C. D., Lindsley, R. C., Carr, S. A. & Ebert, B. L. (2016). "Rps14 haploinsufficiency causes a block in erythroid differentiation mediated by S100A8 and S100A9." *Nat Med*, *22* (3), 288-97. doi: 10.1038/nm.4047.

Schrader, A., Crispatzu, G., Oberbeck, S., Mayer, P., Putzer, S., von Jan, J., Vasyutina, E., Warner, K., Weit, N., Pflug, N., Braun, T., Andersson, E. I., Yadav, B., Riabinska, A., Maurer, B., Ventura Ferreira, M. S., Beier, F., Altmuller, J., Lanasa, M., Herling, C. D., Haferlach, T., Stilgenbauer, S., Hopfinger, G., Peifer, M., Brummendorf, T. H., Nurnberg, P., Elenitoba-Johnson, K. S. J., Zha, S., Hallek, M., Moriggl, R., Reinhardt, H. C., Stern, M. H., Mustjoki, S., Newrzela, S., Frommolt, P. & Herling, M. (2018). "Actionable perturbations of damage responses by TCL1/ATM and epigenetic lesions form the basis of T-PLL." *Nat Commun*, 9 (1), 697. doi: 10.1038/s41467-017-02688-6.

Sebaa, A., Ades, L., Baran-Marzack, F., Mozziconacci, M. J., Penther, D., Dobbelstein, S., Stamatoullas, A., Recher, C., Prebet, T., Moulessehoul, S., Fenaux, P. & Eclache, V. (2012). "Incidence of 17p deletions and TP53 mutation in myelodysplastic syndrome and acute myeloid leukemia with 5q deletion." *Genes Chromosomes Cancer*, 51 (12), 1086-92. doi: 10.1002/gcc.21993.

Seliger, B., Papadileris, S., Vogel, D., Hess, G., Brendel, C., Storkel, S., Ortel, J., Kolbe, K., Huber, C., Huhn, D. & Neubauer, A. (1996). "Analysis of the p53 and MDM-2 gene in acute myeloid leukemia." *Eur J Haematol*, 57 (3), 230-40. doi: 10.1111/j.1600-0609.1996.tb01369.x.

Shah, U. A., Chung, E. Y., Giricz, O., Pradhan, K., Kataoka, K., Gordon-Mitchell, S., Bhagat, T. D., Mai, Y., Wei, Y., Ishida, E., Choudhary, G. S., Joseph, A., Rice, R., Gitego, N., Parrish, C., Bartenstein, M., Goel, S., Mantzaris, I., Shastri, A., Derman, O., Binder, A., Gritsman, K., Kornblum, N., Braunschweig, I., Bhagat, C., Hall, J., Graber, A., Ratner, L., Wang, Y., Ogawa, S., Verma, A., Ye, B. H. & Janakiram, M. (2018). "North American ATLL has a distinct mutational and transcriptional profile and responds to epigenetic therapies." *Blood*, 132 (14), 1507-1518. doi: 10.1182/blood-2018-01-824607.

Shields, B. J., Jackson, J. T., Metcalf, D., Shi, W., Huang, Q., Garnham, A. L., Glaser, S. P., Beck, D., Pimanda, J. E., Bogue, C. W., Smyth, G. K., Alexander, W. S. & McCormack, M. P. (2016). "Acute myeloid leukemia requires Hhex to enable PRC2-mediated epigenetic repression of Cdkn2a." *Genes Dev*, 30 (1), 78-91. doi: 10.1101/gad.268425.115.

Sole, F., Luno, E., Sanzo, C., Espinet, B., Sanz, G. F., Cervera, J., Calasanz, M. J., Cigudosa, J. C., Milla, F., Ribera, J. M., Bureo, E., Marquez, M. L., Arranz, E. & Florensa, L. (2005). "Identification of novel cytogenetic markers with prognostic significance in a series of 968 patients with primary myelodysplastic syndromes." *Haematologica, 90* (9), 1168-78.

Solenthaler, M., Matutes, E., Brito-Babapulle, V., Morilla, R. & Catovsky, D. (2002). "p53 and mdm2 in mantle cell lymphoma in leukemic phase." *Haematologica, 87* (11), 1141-50.

Stengel, A., Kern, W., Haferlach, T., Meggendorfer, M., Fasan, A. & Haferlach, C. (2017). "The impact of TP53 mutations and TP53 deletions on survival varies between AML, ALL, MDS and CLL: an analysis of 3307 cases." *Leukemia, 31* (3), 705-711. doi: 10.1038/leu.2016.263.

Stengel, A., Schnittger, S., Weissmann, S., Kuznia, S., Kern, W., Kohlmann, A., Haferlach, T. & Haferlach, C. (2014). "TP53 mutations occur in 15.7% of ALL and are associated with MYC-rearrangement, low hypodiploidy, and a poor prognosis." *Blood, 124* (2), 251-8. doi: 10.1182/blood-2014-02-558833.

Sun, D., Li, Z., Rew, Y., Gribble, M., Bartberger, M. D., Beck, H. P., Canon, J., Chen, A., Chen, X., Chow, D., Deignan, J., Duquette, J., Eksterowicz, J., Fisher, B., Fox, B. M., Fu, J., Gonzalez, A. Z., Gonzalez-Lopez De Turiso, F., Houze, J. B., Huang, X., Jiang, M., Jin, L., Kayser, F., Liu, J. J., Lo, M. C., Long, A. M., Lucas, B., McGee, L. R., McIntosh, J., Mihalic, J., Oliner, J. D., Osgood, T., Peterson, M. L., Roveto, P., Saiki, A. Y., Shaffer, P., Toteva, M., Wang, Y., Wang, Y. C., Wortman, S., Yakowec, P., Yan, X., Ye, Q., Yu, D., Yu, M., Zhao, X., Zhou, J., Zhu, J., Olson, S. H. & Medina, J. C. (2014). "Discovery of AMG 232, a potent, selective, and orally bioavailable MDM2-p53 inhibitor in clinical development." *J Med Chem, 57* (4), 1454-72. doi: 10.1021/jm401753e.

Sun, G. X., Cao, X. S., Li, Q., Wang, Z., Peng, J. & Lu, C. Q. (2013). "[Significance of miR-155, miR-34a and miR-30a expression in diffuse large B-cell lymphoma]." *Zhonghua Yi Xue Yi Chuan Xue Za Zhi*, *30* (1), 79-83. doi: 10.3760/cma.j.issn.1003-9406.2013.01.019.

Surget, S., Descamps, G., Brosseau, C., Normant, V., Maiga, S., Gomez-Bougie, P., Gouy-Colin, N., Godon, C., Bene, M. C., Moreau, P., Le Gouill, S., Amiot, M. & Pellat-Deceunynck, C. (2014). "RITA (Reactivating p53 and Inducing Tumor Apoptosis) is efficient against TP53abnormal myeloma cells independently of the p53 pathway." *BMC Cancer*, *14*, 437. doi: 10.1186/1471-2407-14-437.

Tabe, Y., Sebasigari, D., Jin, L., Rudelius, M., Davies-Hill, T., Miyake, K., Miida, T., Pittaluga, S. & Raffeld, M. (2009). "MDM2 antagonist nutlin-3 displays antiproliferative and proapoptotic activity in mantle cell lymphoma." *Clin Cancer Res*, *15* (3), 933-42. doi: 10.1158/1078-0432.CCR-08-0399.

Takahashi, K., Patel, K., Bueso-Ramos, C., Zhang, J., Gumbs, C., Jabbour, E., Kadia, T., Andreff, M., Konopleva, M., DiNardo, C., Daver, N., Cortes, J., Estrov, Z., Futreal, A., Kantarjian, H. & Garcia-Manero, G. (2016). "Clinical implications of TP53 mutations in myelodysplastic syndromes treated with hypomethylating agents." *Oncotarget*, *7* (12), 14172-87. doi: 10.18632/oncotarget.7290.

Tanaka, K. (2009). "The proteasome: overview of structure and functions." *Proc Jpn Acad Ser B Phys Biol Sci*, *85* (1), 12-36. doi: 10.2183/pjab.85.12.

Tefferi, A. & Pardanani, A. (2015). "Myeloproliferative Neoplasms: A Contemporary Review." *JAMA Oncol*, *1* (1), 97-105. doi: 10.1001/jamaoncol.2015.89.

Teoh, G., Urashima, M., Ogata, A., Chauhan, D., DeCaprio, J. A., Treon, S. P., Schlossman, R. L. & Anderson, K. C. (1997). "MDM2 protein overexpression promotes proliferation and survival of multiple myeloma cells." *Blood*, *90* (5), 1982-92.

Teoh, P. J., Bi, C., Sintosebastian, C., Tay, L. S., Fonseca, R. & Chng, W. J. (2016). "PRIMA-1 targets the vulnerability of multiple myeloma of deregulated protein homeostasis through the perturbation of ER stress via p73 demethylation." *Oncotarget*, *7* (38), 61806-61819. doi: 10.18632/oncotarget.11241.

Teoh, P. J. & Chng, W. J. (2014). "p53 abnormalities and potential therapeutic targeting in multiple myeloma." *Biomed Res Int, 717919.* doi: 10.1155/2014/717919.

Teoh, P. J., Chung, T. H., Sebastian, S., Choo, S. N., Yan, J., Ng, S. B., Fonseca, R. & Chng, W. J. (2014). "p53 haploinsufficiency and functional abnormalities in multiple myeloma." *Leukemia, 28* (10), 2066-74. doi: 10.1038/leu.2014.102.

Tessoulin, B., Descamps, G., Dousset, C., Amiot, M. & Pellat-Deceunynck, C. (2019). "Targeting Oxidative Stress With Auranofin or Prima-1(Met) to Circumvent p53 or Bax/Bak Deficiency in Myeloma Cells." *Front Oncol, 9,* 128. doi: 10.3389/fonc.2019.00128.

Tessoulin, B., Descamps, G., Moreau, P., Maiga, S., Lode, L., Godon, C., Marionneau-Lambot, S., Oullier, T., Le Gouill, S., Amiot, M. & Pellat-Deceunynck, C. (2014). "PRIMA-1Met induces myeloma cell death independent of p53 by impairing the GSH/ROS balance." *Blood, 124* (10), 1626-36. doi: 10.1182/blood-2014-01-548800.

Tessoulin, B., Eveillard, M., Lok, A., Chiron, D., Moreau, P., Amiot, M., Moreau-Aubry, A., Le Gouill, S. & Pellat-Deceunynck, C. (2017). "p53 dysregulation in B-cell malignancies: More than a single gene in the pathway to hell." *Blood Rev, 31* (4), 251-259. doi: 10.1016/j.blre.2017.03.001.

Tiedemann, R. E., Gonzalez-Paz, N., Kyle, R. A., Santana-Davila, R., Price-Troska, T., Van Wier, S. A., Chng, W. J., Ketterling, R. P., Gertz, M. A., Henderson, K., Greipp, P. R., Dispenzieri, A., Lacy, M. Q., Rajkumar, S. V., Bergsagel, P. L., Stewart, A. K. & Fonseca, R. (2008). "Genetic aberrations and survival in plasma cell leukemia." *Leukemia, 22* (5), 1044-52. doi: 10.1038/leu.2008.4.

Trino, S., De Luca, L., Laurenzana, I., Caivano, A., Del Vecchio, L., Martinelli, G. & Musto, P. (2016). "P53-MDM2 Pathway: Evidences for A New Targeted Therapeutic Approach in B-Acute Lymphoblastic Leukemia." *Front Pharmacol, 7,* 491. doi: 10.3389/fphar.2016.00491.

Trino, S., Iacobucci, I., Erriquez, D., Laurenzana, I., De Luca, L., Ferrari, A., Ghelli Luserna Di Rora, A., Papayannidis, C., Derenzini, E., Simonetti, G., Lonetti, A., Venturi, C., Cattina, F., Ottaviani, E.,

Abbenante, M. C., Russo, D., Perini, G., Musto, P. & Martinelli, G. (2016). "Targeting the p53-MDM2 interaction by the small-molecule MDM2 antagonist Nutlin-3a: a new challenged target therapy in adult Philadelphia positive acute lymphoblastic leukemia patients." *Oncotarget*, 7 (11), 12951-61. doi: 10.18632/oncotarget.7339.

Vasmatzis, G., Johnson, S. H., Knudson, R. A., Ketterling, R. P., Braggio, E., Fonseca, R., Viswanatha, D. S., Law, M. E., Kip, N. S., Ozsan, N., Grebe, S. K., Frederick, L. A., Eckloff, B. W., Thompson, E. A., Kadin, M. E., Milosevic, D., Porcher, J. C., Asmann, Y. W., Smith, D. I., Kovtun, I. V., Ansell, S. M., Dogan, A. & Feldman, A. L. (2012). "Genome-wide analysis reveals recurrent structural abnormalities of TP63 and other p53-related genes in peripheral T-cell lymphomas." *Blood*, 120 (11), 2280-9. doi: 10.1182/blood-2012-03-419937.

Vassilev, L. T., Vu, B. T., Graves, B., Carvajal, D., Podlaski, F., Filipovic, Z., Kong, N., Kammlott, U., Lukacs, C., Klein, C., Fotouhi, N. & Liu, E. A. (2004). "*In Vivo* Activation of the p53 Pathway by Small-Molecule Antagonists of MDM2." *Science*, *303*(5659), 844-8. doi: DOI: 10.1126/science.1092472.

Voropaeva, E. N., Pospelova, T. I., Voevoda, M. I., Maksimov, V. N., Orlov, Y. L. & Seregina, O. B. (2019). "Clinical aspects of TP53 gene inactivation in diffuse large B-cell lymphoma." *BMC Med Genomics*, 12 (Suppl 2), 35. doi: 10.1186/s12920-019-0484-9.

Vu, B., Wovkulich, P., Pizzolato, G., Lovey, A., Ding, Q., Jiang, N., Liu, J. J., Zhao, C., Glenn, K., Wen, Y., Tovar, C., Packman, K., Vassilev, L. & Graves, B. (2013). "Discovery of RG7112: A Small-Molecule MDM2 Inhibitor in Clinical Development." *ACS Med Chem Lett*, 4 (5), 466-9. doi: 10.1021/ml4000657.

Wada, M., Bartram, C. R., Nakamura, H., Hachiya, M., Chen, D. L., Borenstein, J., Miller, C. W., Ludwig, L., Hansen-Hagge, T. E., Ludwig, W. D., et al. (1993). "Analysis of p53 mutations in a large series of lymphoid hematologic malignancies of childhood." *Blood*, 82 (10), 3163-9.

Wagner, A. J., Banerji, U., Mahipal, A., Somaiah, N., Hirsch, H. A., Fancourt, C., Levonas, A., Lam, R., Meister, A., Kemp, R. K., Knox, C.,

Rose, S. & Hong, D. S (2015). "phase I trial of the human double minute 2 (HDM2) inhibitor MK-8242 in patients (pts) with advanced solid tumors." *J Clin Oncol, 33*.

Walker, B. A., Mavrommatis, K., Wardell, C. P., Ashby, T. C., Bauer, M., Davies, F., Rosenthal, A., Wang, H., Qu, P., Hoering, A., Samur, M., Towfic, F., Ortiz, M., Flynt, E., Yu, Z., Yang, Z., Rozelle, D., Obenauer, J., Trotter, M., Auclair, D., Keats, J., Bolli, N., Fulciniti, M., Szalat, R., Moreau, P., Durie, B., Stewart, A. K., Goldschmidt, H., Raab, M. S., Einsele, H., Sonneveld, P., San Miguel, J., Lonial, S., Jackson, G. H., Anderson, K. C., Avet-Loiseau, H., Munshi, N., Thakurta, A. & Morgan, G. (2019). "A high-risk, Double-Hit, group of newly diagnosed myeloma identified by genomic analysis." *Leukemia, 33* (1), 159-170. doi: 10.1038/s41375-018-0196-8.

Wang, X. J., Jeffrey Medeiros, L., Bueso-Ramos, C. E., Tang, G., Wang, S., Oki, Y., Desai, P., Khoury, J. D., Miranda, R. N., Tang, Z., Reddy, N. & Li, S. (2017). "P53 expression correlates with poorer survival and augments the negative prognostic effect of MYC rearrangement, expression or concurrent MYC/BCL2 expression in diffuse large B-cell lymphoma." *Mod Pathol, 30* (2), 194-203. doi: 10.1038/modpathol.2016.178.

Watatani, Y., Sato, Y., Miyoshi, H., Sakamoto, K., Nishida, K., Gion, Y., Nagata, Y., Shiraishi, Y., Chiba, K., Tanaka, H., Zhao, L., Ochi, Y., Takeuchi, Y., Takeda, J., Ueno, H., Kogure, Y., Shiozawa, Y., Kakiuchi, N., Yoshizato, T., Nakagawa, M. M., Nanya, Y., Yoshida, K., Makishima, H., Sanada, M., Sakata-Yanagimoto, M., Chiba, S., Matsuoka, R., Noguchi, M., Hiramoto, N., Ishikawa, T., Kitagawa, J., Nakamura, N., Tsurumi, H., Miyazaki, T., Kito, Y., Miyano, S., Shimoda, K., Takeuchi, K., Ohshima, K., Yoshino, T., Ogawa, S. & Kataoka, K. (2019). "Molecular heterogeneity in peripheral T-cell lymphoma, not otherwise specified revealed by comprehensive genetic profiling." *Leukemia, 33* (12), 2867-2883. doi: 10.1038/s41375-019-0473-1.

Weinhold, N., Ashby, C., Rasche, L., Chavan, S. S., Stein, C., Stephens, O. W., Tytarenko, R., Bauer, M. A., Meissner, T., Deshpande, S., Patel, P.

H., Buzder, T., Molnar, G., Peterson, E. A., van Rhee, F., Zangari, M., Thanendrarajan, S., Schinke, C., Tian, E., Epstein, J., Barlogie, B., Davies, F. E., Heuck, C. J., Walker, B. A. & Morgan, G. J. (2016). "Clonal selection and double-hit events involving tumor suppressor genes underlie relapse in myeloma." *Blood*, *128* (13), 1735-44. doi: 10.1182/blood-2016-06-723007.

Welch, J. S., Petti, A. A., Miller, C. A., Fronick, C. C., O'Laughlin, M., Fulton, R. S., Wilson, R. K., Baty, J. D., Duncavage, E. J., Tandon, B., Lee, Y. S., Wartman, L. D., Uy, G. L., Ghobadi, A., Tomasson, M. H., Pusic, I., Romee, R., Fehniger, T. A., Stockerl-Goldstein, K. E., Vij, R., Oh, S. T., Abboud, C. N., Cashen, A. F., Schroeder, M. A., Jacoby, M. A., Heath, S. E., Luber, K., Janke, M. R., Hantel, A., Khan, N., Sukhanova, M. J., Knoebel, R. W., Stock, W., Graubert, T. A., Walter, M. J., Westervelt, P., Link, D. C., DiPersio, J. F. & Ley, T. J. (2016). "TP53 and Decitabine in Acute Myeloid Leukemia and Myelodysplastic Syndromes." *N Engl J Med*, *375* (21), 2023-2036. doi: 10.1056/NEJMoa1605949.

Whitman, S. P., Maharry, K., Radmacher, M. D., Becker, H., Mrozek, K., Margeson, D., Holland, K. B., Wu, Y. Z., Schwind, S., Metzeler, K. H., Wen, J., Baer, M. R., Powell, B. L., Carter, T. H., Kolitz, J. E., Wetzler, M., Moore, J. O., Stone, R. M., Carroll, A. J., Larson, R. A., Caligiuri, M. A., Marcucci, G. & Bloomfield, C. D. (2010). "FLT3 internal tandem duplication associates with adverse outcome and gene- and microRNA-expression signatures in patients 60 years of age or older with primary cytogenetically normal acute myeloid leukemia: a Cancer and Leukemia Group B study." *Blood*, *116* (18), 3622-6. doi: 10.1182/blood-2010-05-283648.

Wiman, K. G. (2010). "Pharmacological reactivation of mutant p53: from protein structure to the cancer patient." *Oncogene*, *29* (30), 4245-52. doi: 10.1038/onc.2010.188.

Woollard, W. J., Pullabhatla, V., Lorenc, A., Patel, V. M., Butler, R. M., Bayega, A., Begum, N., Bakr, F., Dedhia, K., Fisher, J., Aguilar-Duran, S., Flanagan, C., Ghasemi, A. A., Hoffmann, R. M., Castillo-Mosquera, N., Nuttall, E. A., Paul, A., Roberts, C. A., Solomonidis, E. G., Tarrant,

R., Yoxall, A., Beyers, C. Z., Ferreira, S., Tosi, I., Simpson, M. A., de Rinaldis, E., Mitchell, T. J. & Whittaker, S. J. (2016). "Candidate driver genes involved in genome maintenance and DNA repair in Sezary syndrome." *Blood*, *127* (26), 3387-97. doi: 10.1182/blood-2016-02-699843.

Xia, Y., Fan, L., Wang, L., Gale, R. P., Wang, M., Tian, T., Wu, W., Yu, L., Chen, Y. Y., Xu, W. & Li, J. Y. (2015). "Frequencies of SF3B1, NOTCH1, MYD88, BIRC3 and IGHV mutations and TP53 disruptions in Chinese with chronic lymphocytic leukemia: disparities with Europeans." *Oncotarget*, *6* (7), 5426-34. doi: 10.18632/oncotarget.3101.

Xie, Y., Bulbul, M. A., Ji, L., Inouye, C. M., Groshen, S. G., Tulpule, A., O' Malley, D. P., Wang, E. & Siddiqi, I. N. (2014). "p53 expression is a strong marker of inferior survival in de novo diffuse large B-cell lymphoma and may have enhanced negative effect with MYC coexpression: a single institutional clinicopathologic study." *Am J Clin Pathol*, *141* (4), 593-604. doi: 10.1309/AJCPPHMZ6VHF0WQV.

Xu-Monette, Z. Y., Moller, M. B., Tzankov, A., Montes-Moreno, S., Hu, W., Manyam, G. C., Kristensen, L., Fan, L., Visco, C., Dybkaer, K., Chiu, A., Tam, W., Zu, Y., Bhagat, G., Richards, K. L., Hsi, E. D., Choi, W. W., van Krieken, J. H., Huang, Q., Huh, J., Ai, W., Ponzoni, M., Ferreri, A. J., Wu, L., Zhao, X., Bueso-Ramos, C. E., Wang, S. A., Go, R. S., Li, Y., Winter, J. N., Piris, M. A., Medeiros, L. J. & Young, K. H. (2013). "MDM2 phenotypic and genotypic profiling, respective to TP53 genetic status, in diffuse large B-cell lymphoma patients treated with rituximab-CHOP immunochemotherapy: a report from the International DLBCL Rituximab-CHOP Consortium Program." *Blood*, *122* (15), 2630-40. doi: 10.1182/blood-2012-12-473702.

Xu-Monette, Z. Y., Wu, L., Visco, C., Tai, Y. C., Tzankov, A., Liu, W. M., Montes-Moreno, S., Dybkaer, K., Chiu, A., Orazi, A., Zu, Y., Bhagat, G., Richards, K. L., Hsi, E. D., Zhao, X. F., Choi, W. W., Zhao, X., van Krieken, J. H., Huang, Q., Huh, J., Ai, W., Ponzoni, M., Ferreri, A. J., Zhou, F., Kahl, B. S., Winter, J. N., Xu, W., Li, J., Go, R. S., Li, Y., Piris, M. A., Moller, M. B., Miranda, R. N., Abruzzo, L. V., Medeiros,

L. J. & Young, K. H. (2012). "Mutational profile and prognostic significance of TP53 in diffuse large B-cell lymphoma patients treated with R-CHOP: report from an International DLBCL Rituximab-CHOP Consortium Program Study." *Blood*, *120* (19), 3986-96. doi: 10.1182/blood-2012-05-433334.

Yee, K., Martinelli, G., Vey, N., Dickinson, M. J., Seiter, K., Assouline, S., Drummond, M., Yoon, S., Kasner, M., Lee, J., Kelly, K. R., Blotner, S., Higgins, B., Middleton, S., Nichols, G., Chen, G., Zhong, H., Pierceall, W. E., Zhi, J. & Chen, L. (2014). "Phase 1/1b Study of RG7388, a Potent MDM2 Antagonist, in Acute Myelogenous Leukemia (AML) Patients (Pts)." *Blood Blood*, (2014), 124 (21), 116. (21).

Yu, C. H., Chang, W. T., Jou, S. T., Lin, T. K., Chang, Y. H., Lin, C. Y., Lin, K. H., Lu, M. Y., Chen, S. H., Wu, K. H., Wang, S. C., Chang, H. H., Su, Y. N., Hung, C. C., Lin, D. T., Chen, H. Y. & Yang, Y. L. (2020). "TP53 alterations in relapsed childhood acute lymphoblastic leukemia." *Cancer Sci*, *111* (1), 229-238. doi: 10.1111/cas.14238.

Yu, L., Yu, T. T. & Young, K. H. (2019). "Cross-talk between Myc and p53 in B-cell lymphomas." *Chronic Dis Transl Med*, *5* (3), 139-154. doi: 10.1016/j.cdtm.2019.08.001.

Zhang, L., McGraw, K. L., Sallman, D. A. & List, A. F. (2017). "The role of p53 in myelodysplastic syndromes and acute myeloid leukemia: molecular aspects and clinical implications." *Leuk Lymphoma*, *58* (8), 1777-1790. doi: 10.1080/10428194.2016.1266625.

Zhang, W., Wang, Y. E., Zhang, Y., Leleu, X., Reagan, M., Zhang, Y., Mishima, Y., Glavey, S., Manier, S., Sacco, A., Jiang, B., Roccaro, A. M. & Ghobrial, I. M. (2014). "Global epigenetic regulation of microRNAs in multiple myeloma." *PLoS One*, *9* (10), e110973. doi: 10.1371/journal.pone.0110973.

Zhao, C. Y., Grinkevich, V. V., Nikulenkov, F., Bao, W. & Selivanova, G. (2010). "Rescue of the apoptotic-inducing function of mutant p53 by small molecule RITA." *Cell Cycle*, *9* (9), 1847-55. doi: 10.4161/cc.9.9.11545.

BIOGRAPHICAL SKETCH

Wei Cui

Affiliation: University of Kansas Medical Center

Education: MD and MA

Research and Professional Experience:

- 1992 – 1995 Research Assistant, China Medical University
- 1996 – 1997 Research Assistant, Biochemistry, The University of Kansas
- 1997 – 1999 Research Assistant, Pathology & Laboratory Medicine, The University of Kansas Medical Center
- 1999 – 2001, Postdoctoral Research Associate, Microbiology, Molecular Genetics and Immunology, The University of Kansas Medical Center
- 2001 – 2002 Research Chemist, Great Plain Laboratory
- 2002 – 2005, Research Specialist I, Stowers Institute for Medical Research
- 2010 – 2015, Assistant Professor, Pathology & Laboratory Medicine, The University of Kansas Medical Center
- July 1, 2015 – Present, Associate Professor, Pathology & Laboratory Medicine, The University of Kansas Medical Center
- September 1, 2015 – Present, Medical Director of Clinical Flow Cytometry Laboratory, Pathology & Laboratory Medicine, The University of Kansas Medical Center

Professional Appointments: Associate Professor

Publications from the Last 3 Years:

Alali, Z., Graham, A., Swan, K., Flyckt, R., Falcone, T., Cui, W., Yang, X., Christianson, J. & Nothnick, W. B. (2020). 60S acidic ribosomal protein P1 (RPLP1) is elevated in human endometriotic tissue and in a murine model of endometriosis and is essential for endometriotic epithelial cell survival in vitro. *Molecular human reproduction*, *26*(1), 53-64. 31899515.

Aljubran, F., Graham, A., Cui, W. & Nothnick, W. B. (2020). Increased CXCL12 expression in endometrium of women with abnormal uterine bleeding is post-transcriptionally mediated via miR-23b-3p and is associated with decreased expression of the miR-23b-3p/24-3p/27b-3p cluster. *Fertility & Sterility-Science*, in press.

Boatrighta, C., Walkera, C. M., Donalda, J., Cui, W. & Nagji, A. S. (2020). Incidental dedifferentiated mediastinal liposarcoma on F-18-fluciclovine PET/CT. *Clinical Imaging*, *59*, 21-24. 31715513

Brown, L., Zhang, D. & Cui, W. (2020). Flow Cytometric Immunophenotypic Study of Monocytes and Granulocytes in Myeloid Neoplasms and Reactive Conditions: A Single Institution Experience and Literature Review. *Ann Clin Lab Sci*. 2020 May, *50*(3), 327-332. 32581021.

Gao, L., Saeed, A., Golem, S., Zhang, D., Woodroof, J., McGuirk, J., Ganguly, S., Abhyankar, S., Lin, T. L. & Cui, W. (2020). MYC expression associates with poor survival in patients with acute myeloid leukemia and collaborates with overexpressed p53 in leukemic transformation in patients with myelodysplastic syndrome. *International Journal of Laboratory Hematology*. In press.

Gong, Z., Xu, M. L., Chen, M., Cui, W., Kantarjian, H. M., Cortes, J. E., Zhou, T., Tang, G., Wang, W., Medeiros, L. J. & Hu, S. (2019). Philadelphia chromosome-negative acute leukemia in patients with chronic myeloid leukemia. *American journal of hematology*, *94*(10), E256-E259. 31273842.

Nawabi, A., Garcia, J., Jimenez, A., Turner, S., Olyaee, M., Cui, W., Schmitt, T., Kumer, S., Reintjes, M., Taylor, R., Olson, J. & Nawabi,

N., Nawabi, P. (2017). The presence of donor liver granuloma requiring further workup tovrule out parasitic disease. *Journal of Surgical Case Reports*, *2017*(4), rjx042. PMC5400448, 28458868.

Ni, H., Chao, X., Yang, H., Deng, F., Wang, S., Bai, Q., Qian, H., Cui, Y., Cui, W., Shi, Y., Zong, W. X., Wang, Z., Yang, L. & Ding, W. X. (2019). Dual Roles of mTOR in Regulating Liver Injury and Tumorigenesis in Autophagy Defective Mouse Liver. *Hepatology*. 31095752.

Richardson, A. I., Yin, C. C., Cui, W., Li, N., Medeiros, L. J., Li, L. & Zhang, D. (2019). p53 and β-Catenin Expression Predict Poorer Prognosis in Patients With Anaplastic Large-Cell Lymphoma. *Clinical lymphoma, myeloma & leukemia*, *19*(7), e385-e392. 31078446.

Richardson, A., Zhang, D., Woodroof, J. & Cui, W. (2019). p53 expression in large B-cell lymphomas with MYC extra copies and CD99 expression in large B-cell lymphomas in relation to MYC status. *Human pathology*. 30496802.

Rivas, E., Plapp, F. V. & Cui, W. (2020). Flow Cytometric, Morphologic, and Laboratory Comparative Study in Patients With Leukocytosis and Cytopenia. *Am J Clin Pathol*. 31608361.

Sethapati1, V., Cui, W. & Zhang, D. (2018). Metastatic epithelioid hemangioendothelioma to the bone marrow with associated myelofibrosis is resembling primary myelofibrosis. *J. Modern Human Pathology*, *3*(6), 18-21.

In: p53 　　　　　　　　　　　　　ISBN: 978-1-53618-771-7
Editor: Monte Stevens　　　　　　© 2020 Nova Science Publishers, Inc.

Chapter 2

MECHANISMS AND IMPLICATION OF P53 MUTATION IN CANCER

*Eziafa I. Oduah[1] and Steven R. Grossman[1,2,]**

[1]Division of Hematology, Oncology, and Palliative Care
[2]VCU Massey Cancer Center, Virginia Commonwealth University, Richmond, VA, US

ABSTRACT

Mutation of the *TP53* tumor suppressor gene, encoding the p53 protein, is found in nearly half of all human cancers, and is emerging as a potential therapeutic target. Missense mutant p53, in contrast to wildtype p53, can act as an oncogene, and is characterized by high stability and excess accumulation in cancer cells. Tumors harboring missense mutated p53 are dependent on its high level for its oncogenic functions that drive proliferation, invasion and metastasis. Therefore, the presence of oncogenic p53 mutations portends a poorer prognosis in certain cancers. In this chapter, we will discuss the prevalence of p53 mutation in cancers, as well as important mechanisms underlying the impact of p53 mutations, such as loss of function, dominant negative effect and gain of function. We also discuss the prognostic implications of mutant p53 in select cancer

---

* Corresponding Author's E-mail: steven.grossman@vcuhealth.org.

types and introduce emerging therapeutic approaches targeting this pathway in preclinical and clinical studies.

Keywords: p53 mutant, cancer, gain-of-function, loss of function, dominant negative effect, oncogene, prevalence, prognosis, therapeutic targeting, cancer

INTRODUCTION

p53 is a nuclear protein and transcription factor whose function is to induce cell cycle arrest, DNA repair, apoptosis, senescence, and metabolic alteration in response to multiple cellular stressors [1, 2]. As a tumor suppressor, wildtype p53 responds to DNA damage and other cellular stress by transcriptionally activating tumor suppressor signaling pathways, including cell cycle arrest and DNA damage repair pathways, to maintain genomic integrity [3]. Under normal physiological conditions, wildtype p53 is primarily regulated by the E3 ligase, Murine Double Minute 2 (MDM2) which binds to, and ubiquitinates p53 for proteasome degradation [4]. Later findings pointed to the role of the p300/CBP E4 ubiquitin ligase in maintaining wildtype p53 at low cellular levels in unstressed cells through polyubiquitination and subsequent degradation [5, 6]. Upon cellular stress, however, wildtype p53 becomes activated by posttranslational modifications that disrupt its interaction with MDM2, resulting in accumulation of the protein and transcriptional activation of downstream tumor suppressive target genes [7-9].

Wildtype p53 tumor suppressor function is lost in nearly all human tumors. Genetic losses or mutations at the *TP53* gene locus on chromosome 17 account for loss of p53 tumor suppressor function in about 50% of tumors [2, 10, 11]. Indeed, germline *TP53* mutations are well described in the literature and predispose to several cancers [12-16]. However, somatic *TP53* mutations are more prevalent. These include missense, frameshift and deletions, nonsense and silent mutations [17]. Mutant p53 is now a recognized oncogene as mutations not only lead to loss of tumor suppressor function but can also result in a wide array of emergent oncogenic activities [18, 19]. This chapter will focus on the mechanisms of oncogenicity of mutant p53, survival implications in select cancers, and therapeutic opportunities.

P53 MUTATIONS IN CANCER

Mutant p53 is present in about 50 percent of all cancers [10, 17] and with varying frequency across cancer subtypes (discussed in later sections). Of these, the majority are missense mutations (64%), followed by nonsense (13%) and frameshift (12%), splice (8%) and inframe deletions and fusion mutations (3%) (Figure 1) [20, 21]. As the p53 DNA binding domain is required for transcriptional activation of p53 target genes and p53 tumor suppressor functions, it is a hotspot for both germline and somatic inactivating mutations (Figure 2) [19]. Moreover, p53 mutations are broadly classified into contact and conformational mutants. The former are those in which single amino acids known to physically contact DNA are substituted within the DNA binding doman [22, 23]. In the latter, mutations result in unfolding of the protein and conformational changes that also result in decreased DNA binding [24].

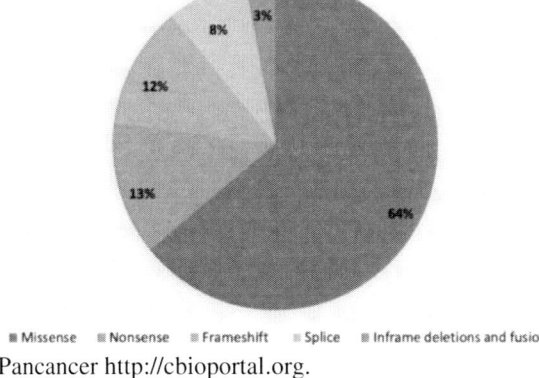

Source; TCGA Pancancer http://cbioportal.org.

Figure 1. Frequency of p53 mutation types.

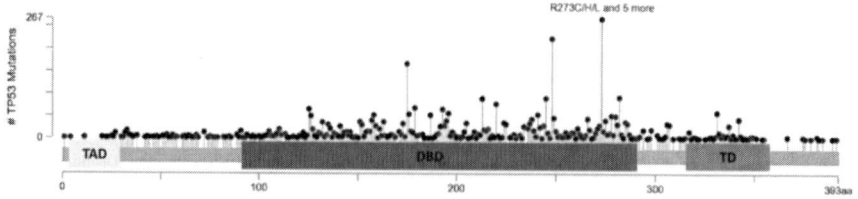

TAD = Transactivation Domain; DBD = DNA Binding Domain; TD = Tetramerization Domain

Source: TCGA Pancancer; http://cbioportal.org/.

Figure 2. Location of mutations on the p53 protein.

Role of *TP53* Mutations in Carcinogenesis

Since p53 plays a central role in maintaining genome integrity, alterations in the p53 pathway are common to almost all cancers either through regulatory or structural abnormalities. Structural alterations, specifically mutations, result in a spectrum of impacts ranging from loss of tumor suppresor function and dominant negative effect (DNE) on the retained wildtype allele to novel oncogenic gain of function (GOF) activities (Figure 3). Indeed, mutant p53 has been implicated in several of the hallmarks of cancer, including sustained proliferation, survival, migration, invasion, metastasis, angiogenesis, genomic instability and altered metabolism [25].

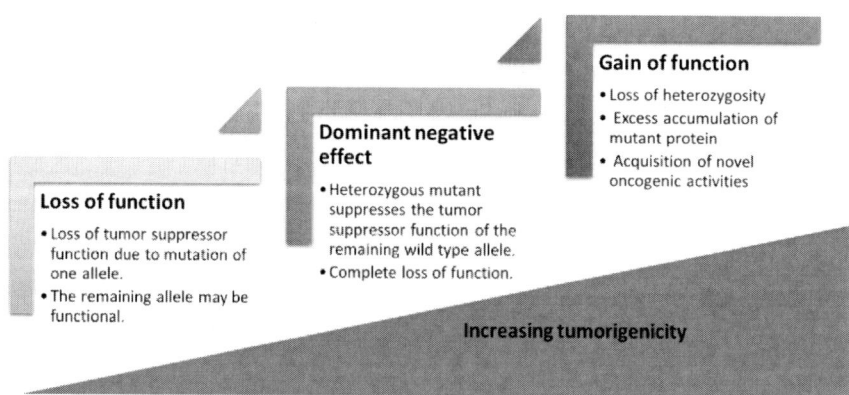

Figure 3. Spectrum of functional implications of p53 mutations.

Loss of Function

Loss of function primarily lies in a deficit in the central function of wild type p53 to maintain genome integrity. The tumor suppressor function of wild type p53 lies in its ability to respond to cellular stress and DNA damage to induce cell cycle arrest, DNA repair, and/or apoptosis [26, 27]. The tumor suppressor function relies on the sequence-specific binding activity of p53 to bind DNA at specific sequences within the promoters of p53 target genes [28, 29]. *TP53* mutations frequently occur in the DNA binding domain (Figure 2), thus impairing its ability to bind the sequences of downstream target genes to induce their transcriptional activation [19]. This results in the inability or delayed ability to arrest the cell cycle, continued proliferation of cells with DNA damage, and propagation of damaged DNA through cellular lineages, leading to genomic instability and malignant clonal selection [1, 31]. All p53 mutations, including nonsense mutations and frameshift deletions, are implicated in p53 loss of function [30].

Dominant Negative Effect

The DNE of mutant p53 describes its ability to inhibit the function of the wildtype protein without confering additional oncogenic properties. Since mutations in *TP53* may occur in only one allele, these mutants may exert inhibitory effects on the wildtype protein, further reducing its tumor suppressor function [1, 31]. In these mutants, complete loss of tumor suppressor function can occur despite heterozygosity of the mutant allele through a mechanism in which the wildtype allele is suppressed by the formation of hetero-oligermers with mutant p53 proteins, inhibiting normal wildtype p53 tetramer formation and subsequent sequence specific DNA binding [1, 32]. Loss of heterozygosity (LOH; loss of the remaining wildtype allele) need not occur [33]. The DNE results in earlier tumor onset and risk of early recurrence compared to cancers where wildtype p53 is not inhibited [34]. Srivasta et al. showed that in cells heterozygous for a missense mutant p53 allele, the mutant allele decreases the transactivation potential of the retained wildtype allele by decreasing binding to wildtype p53-specific transcription factors [35]. Heterozygous mutants also showed delayed transcriptional activation of downstream target genes and defective apoptotic response to ionizing radiation and DNA-damaging agents [36] Other research showed that the DNE resulted in accumulation of the mutant protein and suppression of the anti-oncogenic activity of the wildtype allele without exerting GOF activities [37]. Moreover, the amplitude of these effects are seen in a dose-dependent and cell context dependent manner [38]. A more recent study of isogenic *in vitro* and mouse models of p53 mutants in acute myeloid leukemia (AML) suggested that a DNE was responsible for the phenotypic and functional effects of missense mutations of p53 [31]. The same authors also proposed a model whereby clonal selection of p53 mutants in hematologic malignancies was mediated by the DNE in AML [31].

Gain of Function

The GOF phenotype of mutant p53 is distinct from loss of function and dominant negative phenotypes due to acquisition of novel pro-oncogenic properties by certain mutant p53 aleles. GOF is most commonly seen in missense mutations, but not all p53 mutants acquire these novel oncogenic properties [38]. Important pathophysiologic prerequisites for gain-of-function oncogenicity of mutant p53 have been described, which include stabilization of the mutant protein leading to massive accumulation, activation of pro-oncogenic pathways [39-42], and LOH [43].

The evidence for gain of function originated from mouse stuides that demonstrated increased oncogenicity of p53 mutant tumors compared to p53 null tumors 44-46]. Research since then has further elucidated several manifestations of GOF phenotypes, including early tumor onset [47], a higher propensity for metastasis [42, 48-50], increased invasion [51-53], chemotherapy resistance [53] and radiation resistance [55, 56], inhibition of apoptosis and increased cancer cell survival [57-59], and genomic instability [60, 61]. Early clinical trials also related p53 mutation status to resistance to chemotherapy [62-66].

Several mechanisms have been proposed for the GOF program of mutant p53 and have been previously reviewed [67]. Many of these involve emergent interactions of missense p53 mutants with transcriptional regulators of oncogenic signaling pathways that do not interact with wild type p53. For example, one study showed aberrant cell cycle regulation mediated by the interaction of mutant p53 with NF-Y protien [68, 69]. Vaughan et al. also showed that GOF mutants can interact with and simultaneously transactivate several oncogenic pathways, adding to the complexity of the GOF phenotype [70]. Conversely, mutant p53 can also interact with transcription factors of tumor suppressor pathways to inhibit their function. This is evident from studies of other p53 tumor suppressor family members p63 and p73, in which binding by mutant p53 inhibited their function [71, 72]. In a different study, p53 formed aggregates with tumor suppressors, thus inhibiting their tumor suppressor function [73.

More recent studies have also shown a unique interaction of p53 mutants with the proteasome machinery that drives a GOF program [74]. Yet another sudy showed upregulation of chromatin genes by mutant p53 that results in increased cell proliferation and tumor growth [75]. Mutant GOF p53 also induces and cooperates with proto-oncogenes such as c-Myc that enhance cancer cell survival and proliferation [76, 77]. Frum et al. showed that active DNA damage signaling mediated accumulation of mutant GOF p53, suggesting that constitutive activation of the DNA damage checkpoint may contribute to GOF p53 stabilization and oncogenic signaling [41].

Prognostic Implications of p53 Mutation in Cancers

Mutant p53 is a known indicator of poorer prognosis in several cancers. A query of The Cancer Genome Atlas (TCGA; http://cbioportal.org) supports the findings of individual stuides in several cancer types, showing a statistically significantly poorer overall survival and progression free survival of patients whose tumors express a missense p53 allele. In this section we will discuss evidence supporting the prognostic implications of p53 mutation in select hematologic maligancies and solid tumors.

Hematologic Malignancies

The prevalaence of *TP53* mutations in hemaologic maligancies ranges from 6-30% (Figure 4). p53 mutations are most common in myelodyplatic dysplastic syndromes (MDS) and therapy-related AML. Early studies of

AML, MDS and chronic lymphocytic leukemia (CLL) by Wattel et al. showed that the presence of p53 mutation was a strong indicator of poorer prognosis [78]. A query of TCGA also showed statistically significantly poorer prognosis in hematologic malignancies with p53 mutations (Figure 5).

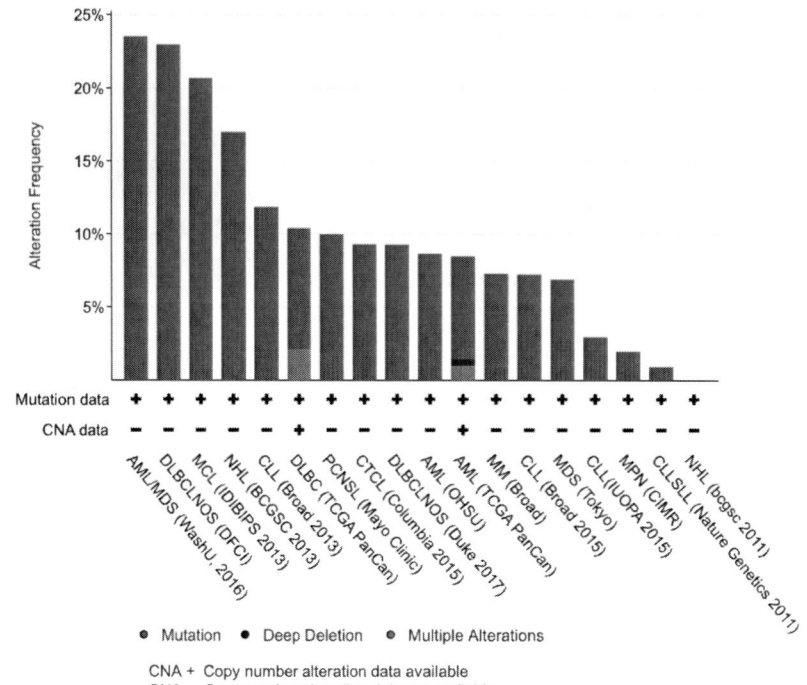

Source: TCGA; http://cbioportal.org/.

Figure 4. Frequency of p53 alterations in hematologic malignancies.

Mechanisms and Implication of p53 Mutation in Cancer

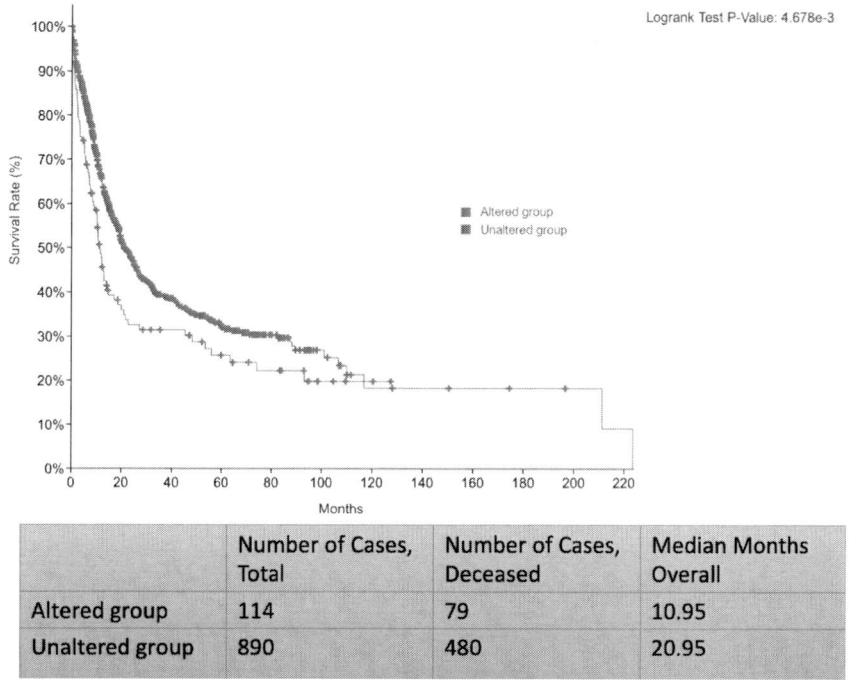

	Number of Cases, Total	Number of Cases, Deceased	Median Months Overall
Altered group	114	79	10.95
Unaltered group	890	480	20.95

Source: TCGA; http://cbioportal.org/.

Figure 5. Overall survival in hematologic malignancies with and without p53 mutation.

TP53 mutations occur in about 6-7% of MDS cases [79-81] but some studies have reported up to 21% [82]. p53 mutations in MDS are known to be associated with complex karyotypes [82] and loss of the remaining wild type allele as indicated by loss of chromosome 17 [81, 82]. Mutant p53 status is an independent prognositic indicator of poorer outcomes in MDS, validated across several studies [80, 81, 83, 84] even after hematopoetic stem cell transplantation [85]. In one study, variant allele frequency (VAF) of the mutation among patients with p53 mutation was a predictor of response and overall survival, such that cases with higher VAF had a poorer prognosis and decreased duration of response [86]. Importantly, the presence of just one mutation was enough to portend poorer prognosis, i.e., the presence of just one mutation was equally significant as the presence of more than one mutation [84].

TP53 is also the most commonly mutated gene in complex karyotype AML and ranks among the top 6 most mutated genes in AML overall [87, 88]. *TP53* mutations are also an established driver mutation in AML, and more common in older patients [89, 90] with close correlation with unfavorable cytogenetic-risk [90] and complex karyotype AML (CK-AML) where the co-occurrence with p53 mutations reaches up to 78% [91]. Although *TP53* mutations occurred less frequently than mutations in genes encoding epigenetic modifiers (*DNM3TA, AXL1, IDH1/2,* and *TET2*), regulators of RNA splicing (*SRSF2, SF3B1, U2AF1, ZRSR2*) and chromatin remodeling (*ASXL1, STAG2, BCOR, MLL, EZH2, PHF6*), mutations in *TP53* remained a significant independent prognostic factor for adverse outcomes with a hazard ratio of 1.7 for death, with negative prognostic impact second only to inv (3) and mutations in *GATA2* and *MECOM*(EVI1), all of which occurred at a much lower frequency than *TP53* mutation [88].

Although the hypomethylating agent azacytadine was previously shown to improve overall survival (OS) compared to conventional care regimens in older patients with AML [92], further subgroup analysis showed that among patients treated with conventional regimens, those with mutated p53 had a significantly decreased overall survival compared to those with wildtype p53 [87]. In another recent study comparing older unfit AML patients with wildtype vs. mutated p53, the investigators found that patients with mutant p53 had a poorer overall survival compared to those who retained wild type p53, despite having similar responses to therapy consisting of the hypomethylating agent decitabine [93].

Among the group of therapy related MDS (t-MDS) and therapy related AML (t-AML) malignancies, p53 mutations are present at a very high frequency of approximately 21 to 40 percent [94, 95]. In spite of the higher frequency of p53 mutations in therapy related diseases compared to *de novo* cases, the mutational spectrum of p53 remains the same [95], with mutations also most frequently occurring within the DNA binding domain. Missense mutations were the most frequent, followed by frameshift and nonsense mutations [95, 96]. As in *de novo* MDS and AML, t-MDS and t-AML also exhibited associated deletions of chromosome 17, indicating LOH and loss of the remaining wild type allele [94]. One study found that de novo AML and MDS mostly carried substitutions at G:C pairs while t- AML and t-MDS had substitutions at A:T pairs [97], though the implication of this is was not emphasized. The presence of p53 mutations in t-MDS and t-AML also portends a dismal prognosis and is an independent indication of poorer overall survival, much worse than de novo cases [95].

Solid Tumors

p53 mutations are more prevalent in solid tumors than in hematologic malignancies (Figure 6). Among solid tumors, p53 mutations occur most frequently in uterine, esophageal, head and neck, lung, and ovarian cancers. The frequency of p53 mutations in these cancers reaches up to 70-90%, depending on histologic subtype. p53 mutation also carries signifcant negative survival implications in solid tumors in a query of the human cancer genome atlas (Figure 7).

Lung Cancer

Somatic *TP53* mutations occur frequently in lung cancer ranging from about 50% in nonsmall cell lung cancer (NSCLC) to 90% in small cell lung cancer (SCLC) [20, 21, 98]. This trend reflects the higher prevalence of p53 mutations in smoking-related lung cancers [99-101]. Several studies have reported that the presence of mutations in p53 connoted a poorer prognosis in lung cancers. In a meta-analysis of studies prior to 2001, the results showed that the presence of mutant p53 was a negative prognostic indicator for all stages of non-small cell lung cancer (NSCLC) (both squamous and adenocarcinoma histologies) [102]. Another study evaluated the impact of p53 overexpression by immunohistochemistry (IHC) and the presence of mutations on survival of NSCLC and response to adjuvant chemotherapy. They found that untreated patients in whom p53 was overexpressed had a poorer prognosis and greater benefit of adjuvant chemotherapy compared to those in whom p53 was undetectable by IHC. However, the presence of mutations alone was neither prognostic nor predictive of response [103]. This finding is interesting in view of the fact that one aforementioned prerequisite for the GOF phenotype is accumulation of p53 to high levels, which makes it detectable by IHC, hence IHC stains have historically been used as a surrogate for the presence of GOF mutation, although it is not a perfect test [104, 105]. Therefore, this finding may point to the suspicion that only those cancers with GOF activities may predict a poorer prognosis from a clinical standpoint.

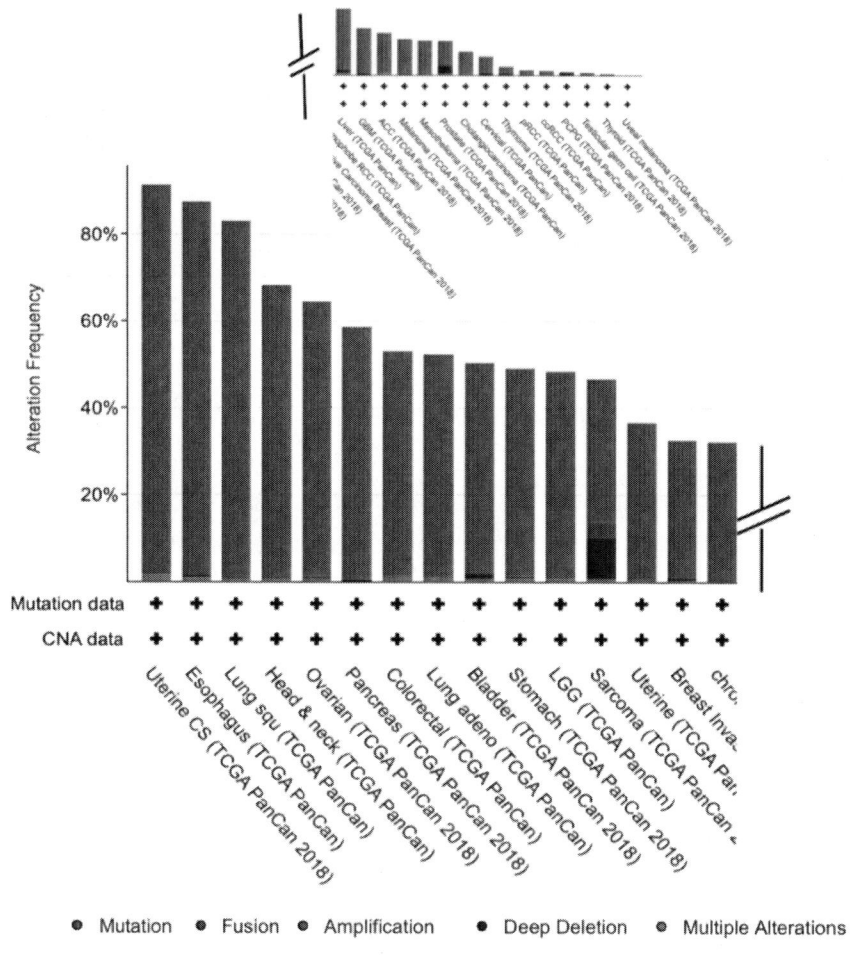

Source: TCGA; http://cbioportal.org.

Figure 6. Frequency of p53 mutations in solid tumors.

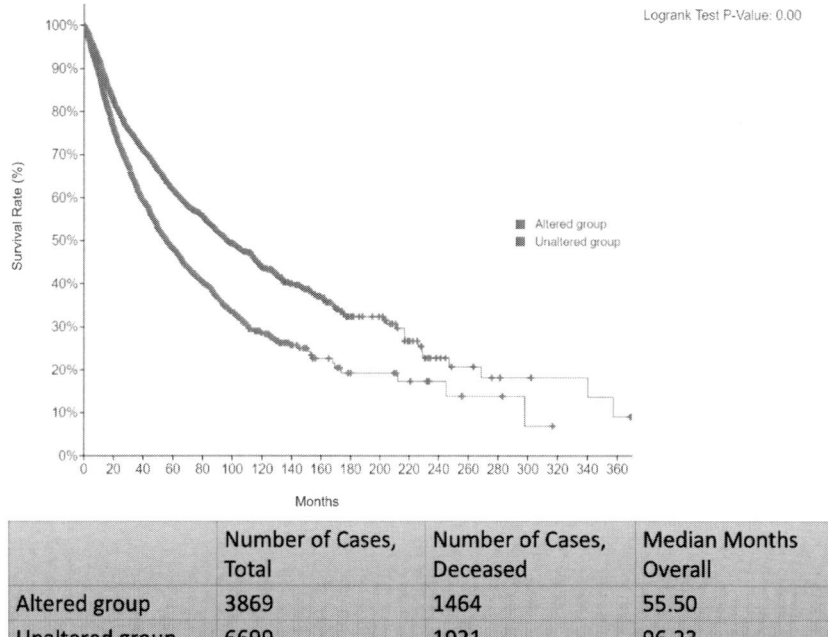

Source: TCGA; http://cbioportal.org/.

Figure 7. Overall survival in solid tumors with and without p53 mutation.

Another meta-analysis of forty-three studies published prior to the year 2000 showed that p53 alteration was a significant marker of poorer prognosis in lung adenocarcinoma but did not reach statistical significance in squamous cell carcinoma of the lung [106]. A more recent meta-analysis of 19 studies up to the year 2015 also evaluated the association of *TP53* mutations in NSCLC. Compared to wildtype p53, mutant p53 bearing cancers had significantly lower overall survival rates [107]. Subgroup analysis showed that the survival benefit of wildtype p53 over mutant p53 was higher in earlier stage cancers and adenocarcinoma, suggesting that the role of mutant p53 may differ depending on disease stage and histological subtype [107].

More recent analyses have focused on the prognostic impact of p53 co-mutations with other driver mutations in lung cancer. These have also consistently shown association with poorer responses to therapy and prognosis within this context. For example, a study of p53 and *ALK* co-mutation in NSCLC showed significantly decreased objective response rate and disease control rate to crizotinib in the presence of *TP53* mutations [108]. In another study, the authors compared the effect of p53 co-mutation in *ALK*-rearranged advanced stage NSCLC in three treatment arms including chemotherapy alone, chemotherapy plus the ALK inhibitor crizotinib or crizotinib plus next generation ALK inhibitor. Their results showed poorer progression free survival and overall survival rates in p53-comutated cases across all treatment arms, compared to those in which wildtype p53 was retained [109].

In another study of *ERBB1* (EGFR) and *TP53* co-mutation, the presence of p53 co-mutation was associated with an inferior overall survival [110]. In the same study, 5.6 percent of patients transformed to small cell cancer. Eighty percent of the transformed cases had p53-comutation. This result is consistent with an even more recent retrospective analysis of a cohort of stage IV NSCLC with EGFR/p53 co-mutations treated with EGFR tyrosine kinase inhibitors. Their analyses revealed that p53 co-mutation was an independent prognostic indicator of poorer overall response rate, disease free survival, and overall survival rates [111].

Ovarian Cancer

TP53 is one of the most frequently mutated genes in high grade serous ovarian cancer, with independent studies showing mutational rates that range from 40-90%, depending on the method of detection and stage of disease [112-114]. One of the early studies suggesting negative prognosis in relation to p53 mutations in human ovarian cancers was performed by Hartman et al. 1994. The authors analyzed p53 status of 284 patients with epithelial ovarian cancer in all 4 stages of the disease by immunohistochemistry. In a univariate analysis, they found that p53 mutation was associated with decreased survival but it did not retain independent prognostic value in a multivariate analysis [115]. Since then, several studies have followed showing decreased time to progression and overall survival as well as resistance to platinum chemotherapy [116-118]. While some studies have suggested poorer prognosis associated with p53 mutations in ovarian cancer, others did not; this was previously reviewed

[119, 120]. Therefore, the overall clinical impact of p53 mutations in ovarian cancer has remained controversial.

Head and Neck Cancer

TP53 mutations occur on over fifty percent of head and neck cancers, with a higher prevalence in patients with a history of smoking and alcohol use [121]. The presence of p53 mutation in head and neck cancer has been associated with poorer response to chemotherapy [122] and poorer overall survival following surgical therapy [123] or radiation therapy [124, 125]. In 2002, Osman et al. compared outcomes in head and neck cancer patients who were treated on a larynx preservation protocol. The presence of greater than twenty percent immunoreactivity for p53 (used as a surrogate marker for p53 mutation and accumulation) had inferior overall survival and worse local disease control [126]. A similar study comparing p53 positive status by immunohistochemistry showed that p53 positivity, used again as a surrogate for the presence of accumulated mutant p53, correlated with a lower recurrence free survival, and lower overall disease specific survival [127]. Despite these, some others have not found a correlation between p53 IHC staining and survival in head and neck cancers. A meta-analysis of studies examining the impact of p53 mutations was inconclusive but highlighted the fact that different studies have used vastly different cutoffs for immunoreactivity, which could have accounted for the inconsistency [128]. Moreover, studies in which mutational analysis was confirmed by RT-PCR were more consistent in correlating the presence of p53 mutations with a poorer overall survival and recurrence [123, 129] suggesting that a more standardized approach to determining p53 status is warranted.

Current Advances and Issues in Therapeutic Targeting of Mutant p53

Given the prevalence and significance of p53 mutations in cancers, p53 mutants are emerging as a potential therapeutic target. Despite ongoing efforts, no therapeutic agent primarily targeting this pathway has had clinical success, as of yet. Available therapeutic strategies to targeting mutant p53 can be broadly categorized mechanistically into direct and indirect targeting approaches (Figure 8): targeting its stability and accumulation; reactivation of wildtype p53; indirect targeting by inducing synthetic lethality or inhibition of downstream effectors.

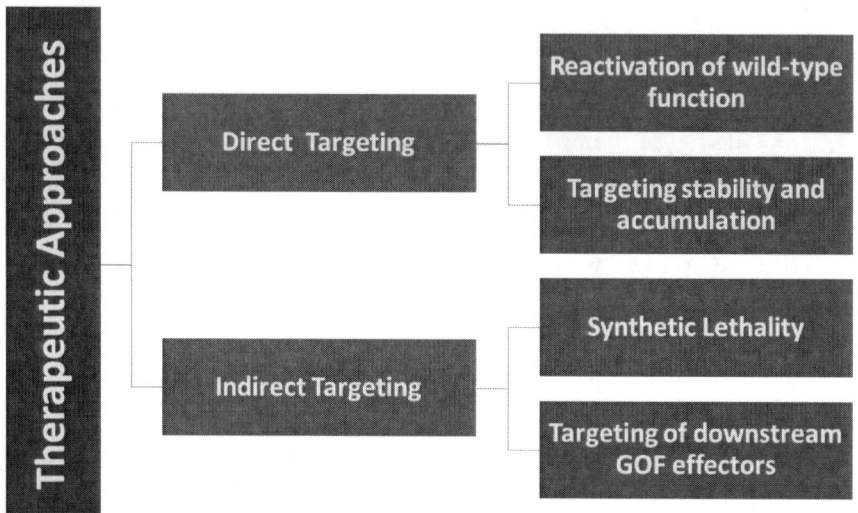

Figure 8. Strategies for therapeutic targeting of mutant p53.

Targeting Mutant p53 Stability and Accumulation

In cancer cells, mutant p53 evades MDM2 dependent degradation and accumulates to excess levels. This is in contrast to untransformed cells, in which mutant p53 does not accumulate, as MDM2 retains its ability to efficiently degrade mutant p53 [39]. Given these observations, it was proposed that other factors within the tumor microenvironment are responsible for the selective advantage of accumulation of GOF p53 [39]. That the excess accumulated mutant p53 exerts GOF activities, renders it a cancer-specific therapeutic target. The evidence for this approach stems from *in vitro* and *in vivo* experiments in which genetic ablation of mutant p53 resulted in induction of apoptosis in cancer cells. and increased survival in mouse models [42, 130].

The Hsp90 chaperone protein was previously shown to regulate mutant p53 conformation and stability [131, 132] Later studies also showed that Hsp90 directly inhibits mutant p53 ubiquitination by inactivating the E3 ligases MDM2 and CHIP [133, 134]. Therefore, using inhibitors of Hsp90, ablation of GOF p53 was seen with therapeutic effect in preclinical studies [135-137]. However, in a recent clinical trial of an Hsp90 inhibitor in p53 mutant ovarian cancer, addition of the Hsp90 inhibitor to paclitaxel showed poorer outcomes than paclitaxel alone [138].

Other studies have also implicated histone deacetylase 6 (HDAC6), a positive regulator of Hsp90, in the accumulation of mutant p53 and showed response to HDAC6 inhibitors in preclinical studies [139, 140]. HDAC6 inhibitors are currently in clinical trials in combination therapy for different cancers. One study in multiple myeloma with available results showed improved response in an HDAC6 inhibitor (Panobinostat) treated arm, but selection was not based on mutant p53 status [141].

Proteasome inhibitors have been shown to cause paradoxical degradation of mutant p53 in *in vitro* studies [142-144], though clinical trials of proteasome inhibitors have not directly addressed the potential for targeting mutant p53 [25].

Arsenic trioxide (ATO), a drug used in acute promyelocytic leukemia, was also described to induce degradation and depletion of mutant p53 through induction of the E3 ligase Pirh2 [145, 146]. Clinical trials are currently ongoing for use of ATO in recurrent and metastatic ovarian and endometrial cancers with p53 mutation, and AML with p53 mutation [147].

Reactvation of Wildtype p53 Function in Mutants

Reactivation of wildtype function for mutant p53 was initially developed as a therapeutic strategy in the 1990s by introduction of second site suppressor mutations to restore DNA binding function [148-151] or by use of synthetic peptides derived from the p53 C-terminus [151]. PRIMA-1 (p53 reactivation and induction of massive apoptosis] was subsequently discovered as a small molecule hit that suppressed mutant p53 cell growth and was found to restore p53 dependent apoptosis in a dose dependent manner [153, 154]. Its structural analog PRIMA-1^{MET} (APR-246) was shown to synergize with chemotherapy [155]. Early phase clinical trials of APR-246 showed promising results in its ability to restore mutant p53 transcriptional activity in human cancers. These studies showed tolerability and some evidence of clinical efficacy in patients with mutant p53 [156, 157]. One multicenter study of APR-246 in ovarian cancer is complete, however the results are currently pending [158].

Synthetic Lethality

Synthetic lethality is a therapeutic approach against GOF p53 in which cell death is induced by targeting GOF p53 dependent pathways [159]. For example, selective upregulation of the platelet derived growth factor receptor β (PDGFRβ) was found to enhance metastasis in a mutant p53 expressing pancreatic cancer model [160]. This upregulation of PDGFRβ was mediated by mutant p53-dependent inhibition of the negative regulator of PDGFRβ, p73/NF-γ complex. Therefore, treatment with the tyrosine kinase inhibitor, imatinib, induced synthetic lethality in these cells. Another example was demonstrated in a clinical trial by Oden-Gangloff et al, where mutant p53 status was shown to significantly correlate to better response to an anti-EGFR-based regimen (cetuximab) [161]. It was thought that this is attributable to crosstalk between EGFR signaling and the p53 pathway [162] and the dependence of GOF p53 driven invasion on EGFR/MEK signaling [163, 164].

Another notable example of the use of synthetic lethality against GOF p53 is the use of CHK1 inhibitors. Cancer cells expressing mutant p53 lack the G1 checkpoint response due to the loss of p21 expression normally induced by wild type p53 in response to DNA damage [165]. These mutant p53 cells are therefore dependent on CHK1 mediated G2 arrest in order to repair DNA after exposure to genotoxins [166]. Moreover, CHK1 was also recently shown to be critical for DNA replication of lung cancer cells specifically expressing a GOF p53 allele, and CHK1 inhibition abrogated proliferation of GOF p53 expressing, but not wild type p53 or p53-null, lung cancer cells [167]. Given the critical roles of CHK1 in both DNA replication and the G2 checkpoint in GOF p53 expressing cancer cells, a number of pre-clinical studies have encouragingly shown that treatment of mutant p53 cancer cells with CHK1 inhibitors in combination with DNA damaging agents results in catastrophic mitosis [168-171].

Other Approaches

In addition to direct targeting of mutant p53, strides have been made towards indirect targeting of this pathway through inhibition of downstream effectors such as metabolic pathways, and oxidative stress [reviewed in 159]. Immunological vaccine targeting of p53 overexpressing cancers was previously reviewed and unfortunately has not progressed past phase I/II studies [172].

CONCLUSION

In summary, the mutant p53 pathway continues to have important implications for cancer progression, treatment resistance and poor prognosis in several cancer types. The emerging landscape of therapeutics targeting this pathway is promising and deserves continued attention. Intelligent design and cross disciplinary collaboration will be important to realize the full potential of targeting this pathway in cancers.

REFERENCES

[1] Lane, D. P. 1992. "p53, Guardian of the Genome." *Nature*. https://doi.org/10.1038/358015a0.

[2] Vousden, Karen H., and Xin Lu. 2002. "Live or Let Die: The Cell's Response to p53." *Nature Reviews Cancer* 2 (8): 594–604. https://doi.org/10.1038/nrc864.

[3] Levine, Arnold J., and Moshe Oren. 2009. "The First 30 Years of p53: Growing Ever More Complex." *Nature Reviews Cancer*. https://doi.org/10.1038/nrc2723.

[4] Momand, Jamil, Gerard P. Zambetti, David C. Olson, Donna George, and Arnold J. Levine. 1992. "The Mdm-2 Oncogene Product Forms a

Complex with the p53 Protein and Inhibits p53-Mediated Transactivation." *Cell* 69 (7): 1237–45. https://doi.org/10.1016/0092-8674(92)90644-R.

[5] Grossman, Steven R., Marco Perez, Andrew L. Kung, Michael Joseph, Claire Mansur, Zhi Xiong Xiao, Sushant Kumar, Peter M. Howley, and David M. Livingston. 1998. "P300/MDM2 Complexes Participate in MDM2-Mediated p53 Degradation." *Molecular Cell* 2 (4): 405–15. https://doi.org/10.1016/S1097-2765(00)80140-9.

[6] Grossman, Steven R., Maria E. Deato, Chrystelle Brignone, Ho Man Chan, Andrew L. Kung, Hideaki Tagami, Yoshihiro Nakatani, and David M. Livingston. 2003. "Polyubiquitination of p53 by a Ubiquitin Ligase Activity of P300." *Science* 300: 342–44. https://doi.org/10.1126/science.1080386.

[7] Shieh, Sheau Yann, Masako Ikeda, Yoichi Taya, and Carol Prives. 1997. "DNA Damage-Induced Phosphorylation of p53 Alleviates Inhibition by MDM2." *Cell* 91 (3): 325–34. https://doi.org/10.1016/S0092-8674(00)80416-X.

[8] Craig, Ashley L., Lindsay Burch, Borek Vojtesek, Jaroslava Mikutowska, Alastair Thompson, and Ted R. Hupp. 1999. "Novel Phosphorylation Sites of Human Tumour Suppressor Protein p53 at Ser20 and Thr18 That Disrupt the Binding of Mdm2 (Mouse Double Minute 2) Protein Are Modified in Human Cancers." *Biochemical Journal* 342 (1): 133–41. https://doi.org/10.1042/0264-6021:3420133.

[9] Appella, Ettore, and Carl W. Anderson. 2001. "Post-Translational Modifications and Activation of p53 by Genotoxic Stresses." *European Journal of Biochemistry.* https://doi.org/10.1046/j.1432-1327.2001.02225.x.

[10] Vogelstein, Bert, David Lane, and Arnold J. Levine. 2000. "Surfing the p53 Network." *Nature* 408 (6810): 307–10. https://doi.org/10.1038/35042675.

[11] Olivier, Magali, Monica Hollstein, and Pierre Hainaut. 2010. "*TP53* Mutations in Human Cancers: Origins, Consequences, and Clinical

Use." *Cold Spring Harbor Perspectives in Biology.* https://doi.org/10.1101/cshperspect.a001008.

[12] Li, F. P., and J. F. Fraumeni. 1969. "Soft-Tissue Sarcomas, Breast Cancer, and Other Neoplasms. A Familial Syndrome?" *Annals of Internal Medicine* 71 (4): 747–52. https://doi.org/10.7326/0003-4819-71-4-747.

[13] Malkin, David, Frederick P. Li, Louise C. Strong, Joseph F. Fraumeni, Camille E. Nelson, David H. Kim, Jayne Kassel, et al. 1990. "Germ Line p53 Mutations in a Familial Syndrome of Breast Cancer, Sarcomas, and Other Neoplasms." *Science* 250 (4985): 1233–38. https://doi.org/10.1126/science.1978757.

[14] Frebourg, T., N. Barbier, Y. X. Yan, J. E. Garber, M. Dreyfus, J. Fraumeni, F. P. Li, and S. H. Friend. 1995. "Germ-Line p53 Mutations in 15 Families with Li-Fraumeni Syndrome." *American Journal of Human Genetics* 56 (3): 608–15.

[15] Evans, Susan C., Betsy Minis, Kelly M. McMasters, Carolyn J. Foster, Mariza DeAndrade, Christopher I. Amos, Louise C. Strong, and Guillermina Lozano. 1998. "Exclusion of a p53 Germline Mutation in a Classic Li-Fraumeni Syndrome Family." *Human Genetics* 102 (6): 681–86. https://doi.org/10.1007/s004390050761.

[16] Olivier, Magali, David E. Goldgar, Nayanta Sodha, Hiroko Ohgaki, Paul Kleihues, Pierre Hainaut, and Rosalind A. Eeles. 2003. "Li-Fraumeni and Related Syndromes: Correlation between Tumor Type, Family Structure, and *TP53* Genotype." *Cancer Research* 63 (20): 6643–50.

[17] Olivier, Magali, Ros Eeles, Monica Hollstein, Mohammed A. Khan, Curtis C. Harris, and Pierre Hainaut. 2002. "The IARC *TP53* Database: New Online Mutation Analysis and Recommendations to Users." *Human Mutation.* https://doi.org/10.1002/humu.10081.

[18] Oren, Moshe, and Varda Rotter. 2010. "Mutant p53 Gain-of-Function in Cancer." *Cold Spring Harbor Perspectives in Biology.* https://doi.org/10.1101/cshperspect.a001107.

[19] Shetzer, Yoav, Alina Molchadsky, and Varda Rotter. 2016. "Oncogenic Mutant p53 Gain of Function Nourishes the Vicious

Cycle of Tumor Development and Cancer Stem-Cell Formation." *Cold Spring Harbor Perspectives in Medicine* 6 (10). https://doi.org/10.1101/cshperspect.a026203.

[20] Cerami, Ethan, Jianjiong Gao, Ugur Dogrusoz, Benjamin E. Gross, Selcuk Onur Sumer, Bülent Arman Aksoy, Anders Jacobsen, et al. 2012. "The CBio Cancer Genomics Portal: An Open Platform for Exploring Multidimensional Cancer Genomics Data." *Cancer Discovery* 2 (5): 401–4. https://doi.org/10.1158/2159-8290.CD-12-0095.

[21] Gao, Jianjiong, Bülent Arman Aksoy, Ugur Dogrusoz, Gideon Dresdner, Benjamin Gross, S. Onur Sumer, Yichao Sun, et al. 2013. "Integrative Analysis of Complex Cancer Genomics and Clinical Profiles Using the CBioPortal." *Science Signaling* 6 (269). https://doi.org/10.1126/scisignal.2004088.

[22] Cho, Yunje, Svetlana Gorina, Philip D. Jeffrey, and Nikola P. Pavletich. 1994. "Crystal Structure of a p53 Tumor Suppressor-DNA Complex: Understanding Tumorigenic Mutations." *Science* 265 (5170): 346–55. https://doi.org/10.1126/science.8023157.

[23] Sigal, A., and V. Rotter. 2000. "Oncogenic Mutations of the p53 Tumor Suppressor: The Demons of the Guardian of the Genome." *Cancer Research* 60 (24):6788-6793.

[24] Bullock, Alex N., Julia Henckel, Brian S. Dedecker, Christopher M. Johnson, Penka V. Nikolova, Mark R. Proctor, David P. Lane, and Alan R. Fersht. 1997. "Thermodynamic Stability of Wild-Type and Mutant p53 Core Domain." *Proceedings of the National Academy of Sciences of the United States of America* 94 (26): 14338–42. https://doi.org/10.1073/pnas.94.26.14338.

[25] Oduah, Eziafa I., and Steven R. Grossman. 2020. "Harnessing the Vulnerabilities of p53 Mutants in Lung Cancer–Focusing on the Proteasome: A New Trick for an Old Foe?" *Cancer Biology and Therapy*. https://doi.org/10.1080/15384047.2019.1702403.

[26] Yonish-Rouach, Elisheva, Dalia Resnftzky, Joseph Lotem, Leo Sachs, Adi Kimchi, and Moshe Oren. 1991. "Wild-Type p53 Induces Apoptosis of Myeloid Leukaemic Cells That Is Inhibited by

Interleukin-6." *Nature* 352 (6333): 345–47. https://doi.org/10.1038/352345a0.

[27] Zilfou, Jack T., and Scott W. Lowe. 2009. "Tumor Suppressive Functions of p53." *Cold Spring Harbor Perspectives in Biology.* https://doi.org/10.1101/cshperspect.a001883.

[28] Kern, Scott E., Kenneth W. Kinzler, Arhur Bruskin, David Jarosz, Paula Friedman, Carol Prives, and Bert Vogelstein. 1991. "Identification of p53 as a Sequence-Specific DNA-Binding Protein." *Science* 252 (5013): 1708–11. https://doi.org/10.1126/science.2047879.

[29] Bargonetti, J., I. Reynisdottir, P. N. Friedman, and C. Prives. 1992. "Site-Specific Binding of Wild-Type p53 to Cellular DNA Is Inhibited by SV40 T Antigen and Mutant p53." *Genes and Development* 6 (10): 1886–98. https://doi.org/10.1101/gad.6.10.1886.

[30] Xu, J., J. Wang, Y. Hu, J. Qian, B. Xu, H. Chen, W. Zou, and J. Y. Fang. 2014. "Unequal Prognostic Potentials of p53 Gain-of-Function Mutations in Human Cancers Associate with Drugmetabolizing Activity." *Cell Death and Disease* 5 (3). https://doi.org/10.1038/cddis.2014.75.

[31] Boettcher, Steffen, Peter G. Miller, Rohan Sharma, Marie McConkey, Matthew Leventhal, Andrei V. Krivtsov, Andrew O. Giacomelli, et al. 2019. "A Dominant-Negative Effect Drives Selection of *TP53* Missense Mutations in Myeloid Malignancies." *Science* 365 (6453): 599–604. https://doi.org/10.1126/science.aax3649.

[32] Sturzbecher, H. W., R. Brain, C. Addison, K. Rudge, M. Remm, M. Grimaldi, E. Keenan, and J. R. Jenkins. 1992. "A C-Terminal α-Helix plus Basic Region Motif Is the Major Structural Determinant of p53 Tetramerization." *Oncogene* 7 (8): 1513–23.

[33] Liu, Yu, Chong Chen, Zhengmin Xu, Claudio Scuoppo, Cory D. Rillahan, Jianjiong Gao, Barbara Spitzer, et al. 2016. "Deletions Linked to *TP53* Loss Drive Cancer through p53-Independent Mechanisms." *Nature* 531 (7595): 471–75. https://doi.org/10.1038/nature17157.

[34] Hassan, Nur Mohammad Monsur, Mitsuhiro Tada, Jun ichi Hamada, Haruhiko Kashiwazaki, Takeshi Kameyama, Rahena Akhter, Yutaka Yamazaki, Masahiro Yano, Nobuo Inoue, and Tetsuya Moriuchi. 2008. "Presence of Dominant Negative Mutation of *TP53* Is a Risk of Early Recurrence in Oral Cancer." *Cancer Letters* 270 (1): 108–19. https://doi.org/10.1016/j.canlet.2008.04.052.

[35] Srivastava, Shiv, Shouwen Wang, Yue Ao Tong, Zheng Mei Hao, and Esther H. Chang. 1993. "Dominant Negative Effect of a Germ-Line Mutant p53: A Step Fostering Tumorigenesis." *Cancer Research* 53 (19): 4452–55.

[36] Vries, Annemieke De, Elsa R. Flores, Barbara Miranda, Harn Mei Hsieh, Conny Th M. Van Oostrom, Julien Sage, and Tyler Jacks. 2002. "Targeted Point Mutations of p53 Lead to Dominant-Negative Inhibition of Wild-Type p53 Function." *Proceedings of the National Academy of Sciences of the United States of America* 99 (5): 2948–53. https://doi.org/10.1073/pnas.052713099.

[37] Hegi, Monika E., Michael A. Klein, Daniela Rüedi, Patrick Chène, Marie France Hamou, and Adriano Aguzzi. 2000. "p53 Transdominance but No Gain of Function in Mouse Brain Tumor Model." *Cancer Research* 60 (11): 3019–24.

[38] Lee, Ming Kei, Wei Wei Teoh, Beng Hooi Phang, Wei Min Tong, Zhao Qi Wang, and Kanaga Sabapathy. 2012. "Cell-Type, Dose, and Mutation-Type Specificity Dictate Mutant p53 Functions In Vivo." *Cancer Cell* 22 (6): 751–64. https://doi.org/10.1016/j.ccr.2012.10.022.

[39] Terzian, Tamara, Young Ah Suh, Tomoo Iwakuma, Sean M. Post, Manja Neumann, Gene A. Lang, Carolyn S. Van Pelt, and Guillermina Lozano. 2008. "The Inherent Instability of Mutant p53 Is Alleviated by Mdm2 or P16 INK4a Loss." *Genes and Development* 22 (10): 1337–44. https://doi.org/10.1101/gad.1662908.

[40] Suh, Young Ah, Sean M. Post, Ana C. Elizondo-Fraire, Daniela R. Maccio, James G. Jackson, Adel K. El-Naggar, Carolyn Van Pelt, Tamara Terzian, and Guillermina Lozano. 2011. "Multiple Stress

Signals Activate Mutant p53 in Vivo." *Cancer Research* 71 (23): 7168–75. https://doi.org/10.1158/0008-5472.CAN-11-0459.

[41] Frum, Rebecca A., Ian M. Love, Priyadarshan K. Damle, Nitai D. Mukhopadhyay, Swati Palit Deb, Sumitra Deb, and Steven R. Grossman. 2016. "Constitutive Activation of DNA Damage Checkpoint Signaling Contributes to Mutant p53 Accumulation via Modulation of p53 Ubiquitination." *Molecular Cancer Research* 14 (5): 423–36. https://doi.org/10.1158/1541-7786.MCR-15-0363.

[42] Alexandrova, E. M., A. R. Yallowitz, D. Li, S. Xu, R. Schulz, D. A. Proia, G. Lozano, M. Dobbelstein, and U. M. Moll. 2015. "Improving Survival by Exploiting Tumour Dependence on Stabilized Mutant p53 for Treatment." *Nature* 523 (7560): 352–56. https://doi.org/10.1038/nature14430.

[43] Alexandrova, Evguenia M., Safia A. Mirza, Sulan Xu, Ramona Schulz-Heddergott, Natalia D. Marchenko, and Ute M. Moll. 2017. "p53 Loss-of-Heterozygosity Is a Necessary Prerequisite for Mutant p53 Stabilization and Gain-of-Function in Vivo." *Cell Death and Disease* 8 (3). https://doi.org/10.1038/cddis.2017.80.

[44] Dittmer, Dirk, Sibani Pati, Gerard Zambetti, Shelley Chu, Angelika K. Teresky, Mary Moore, Cathy Finlay, and Arnold J. Levine. 1993. "Gain of Function Mutations in p53." *Nature Genetics* 4 (1): 42–46. https://doi.org/10.1038/ng0593-42.

[45] Lang, Gene A., Tomoo Iwakuma, Young Ah Suh, Geng Liu, V. Ashutosh Rao, John M. Parant, Yasmine A. Valentin-Vega, et al. 2004. "Gain of Function of a p53 Hot Spot Mutation in a Mouse Model of Li-Fraumeni Syndrome." *Cell* 119 (6): 861–72. https://doi.org/10.1016/j.cell.2004.11.006.

[46] Olive, Kenneth P., David A. Tuveson, Zachary C. Ruhe, Bob Yin, Nicholas A. Willis, Roderick T. Bronson, Denise Crowley, and Tyler Jacks. 2004. "Mutant p53 Gain of Function in Two Mouse Models of Li-Fraumeni Syndrome." *Cell* 119 (6): 847–60. https://doi.org/10.1016/j.cell.2004.11.004.

[47] Hanel, W., N. Marchenko, S. Xu, S. Xiaofeng Yu, W. Weng, and U. Moll. 2013. "Two Hot Spot Mutant p53 Mouse Models Display

Differential Gain of Function in Tumorigenesis." *Cell Death and Differentiation* 20 (7): 898–909. https://doi.org/10.1038/cdd. 2013.17.

[48] Weissmueller, Susann, Eusebio Manchado, Michael Saborowski, John P. Morris IV, Elvin Wagenblast, Carrie A. Davis, Sung Hwan Moon, et al. 2014. "Mutant p53 Drives Pancreatic Cancer Metastasis through Cell-Autonomous PDGF Receptor β Signaling." *Cell* 157 (2): 382–94. https://doi.org/10.1016/j.cell.2014.01.066.

[49] Morton, Jennifer P., Paul Timpson, Saadia A. Karim, Rachel A. Ridgway, Dimitris Athineos, Brendan Doyle, Nigel B. Jamieson, et al. 2010. "Mutant p53 Drives Metastasis and Overcomes Growth Arrest/Senescence in Pancreatic Cancer." *Proceedings of the National Academy of Sciences of the United States of America* 107 (1): 246–51. https://doi.org/10.1073/pnas.0908428107.

[50] Adorno, Maddalena, Michelangelo Cordenonsi, Marco Montagner, Sirio Dupont, Christine Wong, Byron Hann, Aldo Solari, et al. 2009. "A Mutant-p53/Smad Complex Opposes P63 to Empower TGFβ-Induced Metastasis." *Cell* 137 (1): 87–98. https://doi.org/10. 1016/j.cell.2009.01.039.

[51] Muller, Patricia A.J., Patrick T. Caswell, Brendan Doyle, Marcin P. Iwanicki, Ee H. Tan, Saadia Karim, Natalia Lukashchuk, et al. 2009. "Mutant p53 Drives Invasion by Promoting Integrin Recycling." *Cell* 139 (7): 1327–41. https://doi.org/10.1016/j.cell.2009.11.026.

[52] Jiang, W. G., A. J. Sanders, M. Katoh, H. Ungefroren, F. Gieseler, M. Prince, S. K. Thompson, et al. 2015. "Tissue Invasion and Metastasis: Molecular, Biological and Clinical Perspectives." *Seminars in Cancer Biology.* https://doi.org/10.1016/j.semcancer. 2015.03.008.

[53] Nakayama, Mizuho, and Masanobu Oshima. 2019. "Mutant p53 in Colon Cancer." *Journal of Molecular Cell Biology.* https://doi.org/10.1093/jmcb/mjy075.

[54] Zastawny, R. L., R. Salvino, J. Chen, S. Benchimol, and V. Ling. 1993. "The Core Promoter Region of the P-Glycoprotein Gene Is Sufficient to Confer Differential Responsiveness to Wild-Type and Mutant p53." *Oncogene* 8 (6): 1529–35.

[55] Kuerbitz, Steven J., Beverly S. Plunkett, William V. Walsh, and Michael B. Kastan. 1992. "Wild-Type p53 Is a Cell Cycle Checkpoint Determinant Following Irradiation." *Proceedings of the National Academy of Sciences of the United States of America* 89 (16): 7491–95. https://doi.org/10.1073/pnas.89.16.7491.

[56] Lee, J. M., and A. Bernstein. 1993. "p53 Mutations Increase Resistance to Ionizing Radiation." *Proceedings of the National Academy of Sciences of the United States of America* 90 (12): 5742–46. https://doi.org/10.1073/pnas.90.12.5742.

[57] Rusch, Valerie, Nael Martini, David Klimstra, Julie Oliver, Ennapadam Venkatraman, Mark Kris, Ethan Dmitrovsky, et al. 1995. "Aberrant p53 Expression Predicts Clinical Resistance to Cisplatin-Based Chemotherapy in Locally Advanced Non-Small Cell Lung Cancer." *Cancer Research* 55 (21): 5038–42.

[58] Lin, Xinjian, and Stephen B. Howell. 2006. "DNA Mismatch Repair and p53 Function Are Major Determinants of the Rate of Development of Cisplatin Resistance." *Molecular Cancer Therapeutics* 5 (5): 1239–47. https://doi.org/10.1158/1535-7163. MCT-05-0491.

[59] Wang, Xiang, Jin Xiu Chen, Yan Hui Liu, Chao You, and Qing Mao. 2013. "Mutant *TP53* Enhances the Resistance of Glioblastoma Cells to Temozolomide by Up-Regulating O6-Methylguanine DNA-Methyltransferase." *Neurological Sciences* 34 (8): 1421–28. https://doi.org/10.1007/s10072-012-1257-9.

[60] Liu, D. P., H. Song, and Y. Xu. 2010. "A Common Gain of Function of p53 Cancer Mutants in Inducing Genetic Instability." *Oncogene* 29 (7). https://doi.org/10.1038/onc.2009.376.

[61] Song, Hoseok, Monica Hollstein, and Yang Xu. 2007. "p53 Gain-of-Function Cancer Mutants Induce Genetic Instability by Inactivating ATM." *Nature Cell Biology* 9 (5): 573–80. https://doi.org/10.1038/ncb1571.

[62] Horio, Yoshitsugu, Takashi Takahashi, Tetsuo Kuroishi, Kenji Hibi, Motokazu Suyama, Takao Niimi, Kaoru Shimokata, et al. 1993. "Prognostic Significance of p53 Mutations and 3p Deletions in

Primary Resected Non-Small Cell Lung Cancer." *Cancer Research* 53 (1): 1–4.

[63] Bergh, Jonas, Torbjörn Norberg, Sigrid Sjögren, Anders Lindgren, and Lars Holmberg. 1995. "Complete Sequencing of the p53 Gene Provides Prognostic Information in Breast Cancer Patients, Particularly in Relation to Adjuvant Systemic Therapy and Radiotherapy." *Nature Medicine* 1 (10): 1029–34. https://doi.org/10.1038/nm1095-1029.

[64] Aas, Turid, Anne Lise Børresen, Stephanie Geisler, Birgitte Smith-Sørensen, Hilde Johnsen, Jan E. Varhaug, Lars A. Akslen, and Per E. Lønning. 1996. "Specific p53 Mutations Are Associated with de Novo Resistance to Doxorubicin in Breast Cancer Patients." *Nature Medicine* 2 (7): 811–14. https://doi.org/10.1038/nm0796-811.

[65] Hamada, Madoka, Toshiyoshi Fujiwara, Akio Hizuta, Akira Gochi, Yoshio Naomoto, Norihisa Takakura, Kenji Takahashi, Jack A. Roth, Noriaki Tanaka, and Kunzo Orita. 1996. "The p53 Gene Is a Potent Determinant of Chemosensitivity and Radiosensitivity in Gastric and Colorectal Cancers." *Journal of Cancer Research and Clinical Oncology* 122 (6): 360–65. https://doi.org/10.1007/ BF01220804.

[66] Shelling, A. N. 1997. "Role of p53 in Drug Resistance in Ovarian Cancer." *Lancet*. https://doi.org/10.1016/S0140-6736(05)60195-X.

[67] Muller, Patricia A. J., and Karen H. Vousden. 2013. "p53 Mutations in Cancer." *Nature Cell Biology*. https://doi.org/10.1038/ncb2641.

[68] Di Agostino, Silvia, Sabrina Strano, Velia Emiliozzi, Valentina Zerbini, Marcella Mottolese, Ada Sacchi, Giovanni Blandino, and Giulia Piaggio. 2006. "Gain of Function of Mutant p53: The Mutant p53/NF-Y Protein Complex Reveals an Aberrant Transcriptional Mechanism of Cell Cycle Regulation." *Cancer Cell* 10 (3): 191–202. https://doi.org/10.1016/j.ccr.2006.08.013.

[69] Liu, K., S. Ling, and W.-C. Lin. 2011. "TopBP1 Mediates Mutant p53 Gain of Function through NF-Y and P63/P73." *Molecular and Cellular Biology* 31 (22): 4464–81. https://doi.org/10.1128/mcb.05574-11.

[70] Vaughan, Catherine A., Shilpa Singh, Steven R. Grossman, Brad Windle, Swati Palit Deb, and Sumitra Deb. 2017. "Gain-of-Function p53 Activates Multiple Signaling Pathways to Induce Oncogenicity in Lung Cancer Cells." *Molecular Oncology* 11 (6): 696–711. https://doi.org/10.1002/1878-0261.12068.

[71] Strano, Sabrina, Giulia Fontemaggi, Antonio Costanzo, Maria Giulia Rizzo, Olimpia Monti, Alessia Baccarini, Giannino Del Sal, et al. 2002. "Physical Interaction with Human Tumor-Derived p53 Mutants Inhibits P63 Activities." *Journal of Biological Chemistry* 277 (21): 18817–26. https://doi.org/10.1074/jbc.M201405200.

[72] Gaiddon, C., M. Lokshin, J. Ahn, T. Zhang, and C. Prives. 2001. "A Subset of Tumor-Derived Mutant Forms of p53 Down-Regulate P63 and P73 through a Direct Interaction with the p53 Core Domain." *Molecular and Cellular Biology* 21 (5): 1874–87. https://doi.org/10.1128/mcb.21.5.1874-1887.2001.

[73] Xu, Jie, Joke Reumers, José R. Couceiro, Frederik De Smet, Rodrigo Gallardo, Stanislav Rudyak, Ann Cornelis, et al. 2011. "Gain of Function of Mutant p53 by Coaggregation with Multiple Tumor Suppressors." *Nature Chemical Biology* 7 (5): 285–95. https://doi.org/10.1038/nchembio.546.

[74] Walerych, Dawid, Kamil Lisek, Roberta Sommaggio, Silvano Piazza, Yari Ciani, Emiliano Dalla, Katarzyna Rajkowska, et al. 2016. "Proteasome Machinery Is Instrumental in a Common Gain-of-Function Program of the p53 Missense Mutants in Cancer." *Nature Cell Biology* 18 (8): 897–909. https://doi.org/10.1038/ncb3380.

[75] Zhu, Jiajun, Morgan A. Sammons, Greg Donahue, Zhixun Dou, Masoud Vedadi, Matthaus Getlik, Dalia Barsyte-Lovejoy, et al. 2015. "Gain-of-Function p53 Mutants Co-Opt Chromatin Pathways to Drive Cancer Growth." *Nature* 525 (7568): 206–11. https://doi.org/10.1038/nature15251.

[76] Liao, Peng, Shelya X. Zeng, Xiang Zhou, Tianjian Chen, Fen Zhou, Bo Cao, Ji Hoon Jung, Giannino Del Sal, Shiwen Luo, and Hua Lu. 2017. "Mutant p53 Gains Its Function via C-Myc Activation upon CDK4 Phosphorylation at Serine 249 and Consequent PIN1

Binding." *Molecular Cell* 68 (6): 1134-1146.e6. https://doi.org/10.1016/j.molcel.2017.11.006.

[77] Wang, Huai, Peng Liao, Shelya X. Zeng, and Hua Lu. 2019. "It Takes a Team: A Gain-of-Function Story of p53-R249S." *Journal of Molecular Cell Biology*. https://doi.org/10.1093/jmcb/mjy086.

[78] Wattel, Eric, Claude Preudhomme, Bernard Hecquet, Michael Vanrumbeke, Bruno Quesnel, Isabelle Dervite, Pierre Morel, and Pierre Fenaux. 1994. "p53 Mutations Are Associated with Resistance to Chemotherapy and Short Survival in Hematologic Malignancies." *Blood* 84 (9): 3148–57. https://doi.org/10.1182/ blood.v84.9.3148.bloodjournal8493148.

[79] Haferlach, T., Y. Nagata, V. Grossmann, Y. Okuno, U. Bacher, G. Nagae, S. Schnittger, et al. 2014. "Landscape of Genetic Lesions in 944 Patients with Myelodysplastic Syndromes." *Leukemia* 28 (2): 241–47. https://doi.org/10.1038/leu.2013.336.

[80] Papaemmanuil, Elli, Moritz Gerstung, Luca Malcovati, Sudhir Tauro, Gunes Gundem, Peter Van Loo, Chris J. Yoon, et al. 2013. "Clinical and Biological Implications of Driver Mutations in Myelodysplastic Syndromes." *Blood* 122 (22): 3616–27. https://doi.org/10.1182/blood-2013-08-518886.

[81] Bejar, Rafael, Kristen Stevenson, Omar Abdel-Wahab, Naomi Galili, Björn Nilsson, Guillermo Garcia-Manero, Hagop Kantarjian, et al. 2011. "Clinical Effect of Point Mutations in Myelodysplastic Syndromes." *New England Journal of Medicine* 364 (26): 2496–2506. https://doi.org/10.1056/NEJMoa1013343.

[82] Bejar, Rafael, Kristen E. Stevenson, Bennett Caughey, R. Coleman Lindsley, Brenton G. Mar, Petar Stojanov, Gad Getz, et al. 2014. "Somatic Mutations Predict Poor Outcome in Patients with Myelodysplastic Syndrome after Hematopoietic Stem-Cell Transplantation." *Journal of Clinical Oncology* 32 (25): 2691–98. https://doi.org/10.1200/JCO.2013.52.3381.

[83] Bejar, Rafael, Kristen E. Stevenson, Bennett A. Caughey, Omar Abdel-Wahab, David P. Steensma, Naomi Galili, Azra Raza, et al. 2012. "Validation of a Prognostic Model and the Impact of Mutations

in Patients with Lower-Risk Myelodysplastic Syndromes." *Journal of Clinical Oncology* 30 (27): 3376–82. https://doi.org/10.1200/JCO.2011.40.7379.

[84] Montalban-Bravo, Guillermo, Rashmi Kanagal-Shamanna, Christopher B. Benton, Caleb A. Class, Kelly S. Chien, Koji Sasaki, Kiran Naqvi, et al. 2020. "Genomic Context and *TP53* Allele Frequency Define Clinical Outcomes in *TP53*-Mutated Myelodysplastic Syndromes." *Blood Advances* 4 (3): 482–95. https://doi.org/10.1182/bloodadvances.2019001101.

[85] Kharfan-Dabaja, Mohamed A., Rami S. Komrokji, Qing Zhang, Ambuj Kumar, Athanasios Tsalatsanis, Janelle Perkins, Taiga Nishihori, et al. 2017. "*TP53* and IDH2 Somatic Mutations Are Associated With Inferior Overall Survival After Allogeneic Hematopoietic Cell Transplantation for Myelodysplastic Syndrome." *Clinical Lymphoma, Myeloma and Leukemia* 17 (11): 753–58. https://doi.org/10.1016/j.clml.2017.06.003.

[86] Sallman, D. A., R. Komrokji, C. Vaupel, T. Cluzeau, S. M. Geyer, K. L. McGraw, N. H. Al Ali, et al. 2016. "Impact of *TP53* Mutation Variant Allele Frequency on Phenotype and Outcomes in Myelodysplastic Syndromes." *Leukemia* 30 (3): 666–73. https://doi.org/10.1038/leu.2015.304.

[87] Döhner, Hartmut, Anna Dolnik, Lin Tang, John F. Seymour, Mark D. Minden, Richard M. Stone, Teresa Bernal del Castillo, et al. 2018. "Cytogenetics and Gene Mutations Influence Survival in Older Patients with Acute Myeloid Leukemia Treated with Azacitidine or Conventional Care." *Leukemia* 32 (12): 2546–57. https://doi.org/10.1038/s41375-018-0257-z.

[88] Rücker, Frank G., Richard F. Schlenk, Lars Bullinger, Sabine Kayser, Veronica Teleanu, Helena Kett, Marianne Habdank, et al. 2012. "*TP53* Alterations in Acute Myeloid Leukemia with Complex Karyotype Correlate with Specific Copy Number Alterations, Monosomal Karyotype, and Dismal Outcome." *Blood* 119 (9): 2114–21. https://doi.org/10.1182/blood-2011-08-375758.

[89] Papaemmanuil, Elli, Moritz Gerstung, Lars Bullinger, Verena I. Gaidzik, Peter Paschka, Nicola D. Roberts, Nicola E. Potter, et al. 2016. "Genomic Classification and Prognosis in Acute Myeloid Leukemia." *New England Journal of Medicine* 374 (23): 2209–21. https://doi.org/10.1056/NEJMoa1516192.

[90] Ley, Timothy J., Christopher Miller, Li Ding, Benjamin J. Raphael, Andrew J. Mungall, Gordon Robertson, Katherine Hoadley, et al. 2013. "Genomic and Epigenomic Landscapes of Adult de Novo Acute Myeloid Leukemia." *New England Journal of Medicine* 368 (22): 2059–74. https://doi.org/10.1056/NEJMoa1301689.

[91] Bally, Cecile, Lionel Adès, Aline Renneville, Marie Sebert, Virginie Eclache, Claude Preudhomme, Marie Joelle Mozziconacci, Hugues de The, Jacqueline Lehmann-Che, and Pierre Fenaux. 2014. "Prognostic Value of *TP53* Gene Mutations in Myelodysplastic Syndromes and Acute Myeloid Leukemia Treated with Azacitidine." *Leukemia Research* 38 (7): 751–55. https://doi.org/10.1016/j.leukres.2014.03.012.

[92] Dombret, Hervé, John F. Seymour, Aleksandra Butrym, Agnieszka Wierzbowska, Dominik Selleslag, Jun Ho Jang, Rajat Kumar, et al. 2015. "International Phase 3 Study of Azacitidine vs Conventional Care Regimens in Older Patients with Newly Diagnosed AML with >30% Blasts." *Blood* 126 (3): 291–99. https://doi.org/10.1182/ blood-2015-01-621664.

[93] Becker, Heiko, Dietmar Pfeifer, Gabriele Ihorst, Milena Pantic, Julius Wehrle, Björn H. Rüter, Lars Bullinger, et al. 2020. "Monosomal Karyotype and Chromosome 17p Loss or *TP53* Mutations in Decitabine-Treated Patients with Acute Myeloid Leukemia." *Annals of Hematology* 99 (7): 1551–60. https://doi.org/ 10.1007/s00277-020-04082-7.

[94] Shih, Alan H., Stephen S. Chung, Emily K. Dolezal, Su Jiang Zhang, Omar I. Abdel-Wahab, Christopher Y. Park, Stephen D. Nimer, Ross L. Levine, and Virginia M. Klimek. 2013. "Mutational Analysis of Therapy-Related Myelodysplastic Syndromes and Acute

Myelogenous Leukemia." *Haematologica* 98 (6): 908–12. https://doi.org/10.3324/haematol.2012.076729.

[95] Ok, Chi Young, Keyur P. Patel, Guillermo Garcia-Manero, Mark J. Routbort, Jie Peng, Guilin Tang, Maitrayee Goswami, et al. 2015. "*TP53* Mutation Characteristics in Therapy-Related Myelodysplastic Syndromes and Acute Myeloid Leukemia Is Similar to de Novo Diseases." *Journal of Hematology and Oncology* 8 (1). https://doi.org/10.1186/s13045-015-0139-z.

[96] Wong, Terrence N., Giridharan Ramsingh, Andrew L. Young, Christopher A. Miller, Waseem Touma, John S. Welch, Tamara L. Lamprecht, et al. 2015. "Role of *TP53* Mutations in the Origin and Evolution of Therapy-Related Acute Myeloid Leukaemia." *Nature* 518 (7540): 552–55. https://doi.org/10.1038/nature13968.

[97] Christiansen, D. H., M. K. Andersen, and J. Pedersen-Bjergaard. 2001. "Mutations with Loss of Heterozygosity of p53 Are Common in Therapy-Related Myelodysplasia and Acute Myeloid Leukemia after Exposure to Alkylating Agents and Significantly Associated with Deletion or Loss of 5q, a Complex Karyotype, and a Poor Prognosis." *Journal of Clinical Oncology* 19 (5): 1405–13. https://doi.org/10.1200/JCO.2001.19.5.1405.

[98] Peifer, Martin, Lynnette Fernández-Cuesta, Martin L. Sos, Julie George, Danila Seidel, Lawryn H. Kasper, Dennis Plenker, et al. 2012. "Integrative Genome Analyses Identify Key Somatic Driver Mutations of Small-Cell Lung Cancer." *Nature Genetics* 44 (10): 1104–10. https://doi.org/10.1038/ng.2396.

[99] Husgafvel-Pursiainen, Kirsti, Paolo Boffetta, Annamaria Kannio, Fredrik Nyberg, Göran Pershagen, Anush Mukeria, Vali Constantinescu, Cristina Fortes, and Simone Benhamou. 2000. "p53 Mutations and Exposure to Environmental Tobacco Smoke in a Multicenter Study on Lung Cancer." *Cancer Research* 60 (11): 2906–11.

[100] Takagi, Y., H. Osada, T. Kuroishi, T. Mitsudomi, M. Kondo, T. Niimi, S. Saji, et al. 1998. "p53 Mutations in Non-Small-Cell Lung Cancers Occurring in Individuals without a Past History of Active

Smoking." *British Journal of Cancer* 77 (10): 1568–72. https://doi.org/10.1038/bjc.1998.258.

[101] Hainaut, Pierre, Magali Olivier, and Gerd P. Pfeifer. 2001. "*TP53* Mutation Spectrum in Lung Cancers and Mutagenic Signature of Compenents of Tobacco Smoke: Lessons from the IARC *TP53* Mutation Database [1]." *Mutagenesis*. https://doi.org/10.1093/mutage/16.6.551.

[102] Steels, E., M. Paesmans, T. Berghmans, F. Branle, F. Lemaitre, C. Mascaux, A. P. Meert, F. Vallot, J. J. Lafitte, and J. P. Sculier. 2001. "Role of p53 as a Prognostic Factor for Survival in Lung Cancer: A Systematic Review of the Literature with a Meta-Analysis." *European Respiratory Journal* 18 (4): 705–19. https://doi.org/10.1183/09031936.01.00062201.

[103] Tsao, Ming Sound, Sarit Aviel-Ronen, Keyue Ding, Davina Lau, Ni Liu, Akira Sakurada, Marlo Whitehead, et al. 2007. "Prognostic and Predictive Importance of p53 and RAS for Adjuvant Chemotherapy in Non-Small-Cell Lung Cancer." *Journal of Clinical Oncology* 25 (33): 5240–47. https://doi.org/10.1200/JCO.2007.12.6953.

[104] Iggo, R., J. Bartek, D. Lane, K. Gatter, A. L. Harris, and J. Bartek. 1990. "Increased Expression of Mutant Forms of p53 Oncogene in Primary Lung Cancer." *The Lancet* 335 (8691): 675–79. https://doi.org/10.1016/0140-6736(90)90801-B.

[105] Dubinski, William, Natasha B. Leighl, Ming Sound Tsao, and David M. Hwang. 2012. "Ancillary Testing in Lung Cancer Diagnosis." *Pulmonary Medicine*. https://doi.org/10.1155/2012/249082.

[106] Mitsudomi, T., N. Hamajima, M. Ogawa, and T. Takahashi. 2000. "Prognostic Significance of p53 Alterations in Patients with Non-Small Cell Lung Cancer: A Meta-Analysis." *Clinical Cancer Research* 6 (10).

[107] Gu, Jincui, Yanbin Zhou, Lixia Huang, Weijun Ou, Jian Wu, Shaoli Li, Junwen Xu, Jinlun Feng, and Baomo Liu. 2016. "*TP53* Mutation Is Associated with a Poor Clinical Outcome for Non-Small Cell Lung Cancer: Evidence from a Meta-Analysis." *Molecular and Clinical Oncology* 5 (6): 705–13. https://doi.org/10.3892/mco.2016.1057.

[108] Song, Peng, Fanshuang Zhang, Yan Li, Guangjian Yang, Wenbin Li, Jianming Ying, and Shugeng Gao. 2019. "Concomitant *TP53* Mutations with Response to Crizotinib Treatment in Patients with ALK-Rearranged Non-Small-Cell Lung Cancer." *Cancer Medicine* 8 (4): 1551–57. https://doi.org/10.1002/cam4.2043.

[109] Kron, A., C. Alidousty, M. Scheffler, S. Merkelbach-Bruse, D. Seidel, R. Riedel, M. A. Ihle, et al. 2018. "Impact of *TP53* Mutation Status on Systemic Treatment Outcome in ALK-Rearranged Non-Small-Cell Lung Cancer." *Annals of Oncology* 29 (10): 2068–75. https://doi.org/10.1093/annonc/mdy333.

[110] Aggarwal, Charu, Christiana W. Davis, Rosemarie Mick, Jeffrey C. Thompson, Saman Ahmed, Seth Jeffries, Stephen Bagley, et al. 2018. "Influence of *TP53* Mutation on Survival in Patients With Advanced EGFR -Mutant Non–Small-Cell Lung Cancer." *JCO Precision Oncology*, no. 2: 1–29. https://doi.org/10.1200/po.18. 00107.

[111] Roeper, Julia, Markus Falk, Athena Chalaris-Rißmann, Anne C. Lueers, Hayat Ramdani, Katrin Wedeken, Ursula Stropiep, et al. 2020. "*TP53* Co-Mutations in EGFR Mutated Patients in NSCLC Stage IV: A Strong Predictive Factor of ORR, PFS and OS in EGFR Mt+ NSCLC." *Oncotarget* 11 (3): 250–64. https://doi.org/10.18632/oncotarget.27430.

[112] Schuijer, Monique, and Els M. J. J. Berns. 2003. "*TP53* and Ovarian Cancer." *Human Mutation*. https://doi.org/10.1002/humu.10181.

[113] Berns, Els M. J. J., and David D. Bowtell. 2012. "The Changing View of High-Grade Serous Ovarian Cancer." *Cancer Research*. https://doi.org/10.1158/0008-5472.CAN-11-3911.

[114] Bell, D., A. Berchuck, M. Birrer, J. Chien, D. W. Cramer, F. Dao, R. Dhir, et al. 2011. "Integrated Genomic Analyses of Ovarian Carcinoma." *Nature* 474 (7353): 609–15. https://doi.org/10.1038/nature10166.

[115] Hartmann, Lynn C., Karl C. Podratz, Gary L. Keeney, Nermeen A. Kamel, John H. Edmonson, Joseph P. Grill, John Q. Su, Jerry A. Katzmann, and Patrick C. Roche. 1994. "Prognostic Significance of p53 Immunostaining in Epithelial Ovarian Cancer." *Journal of*

Clinical Oncology 12 (1): 64–69. https://doi.org/10.1200/JCO.1994.12.1.64.

[116] Herod, J. Jonathan O., Aristides G. Eliopoulos, Jane Warwick, Gerald Niedobitek, Lawrence S. Young, and David J. Kerr. 1996. "The Prognostic Significance of Bcl-2 and p53 Expression in Ovarian Carcinoma." *Cancer Research* 56 (9): 2178–84.

[117] Buttitta, F., A. Marchetti, A. Gadducci, S. Pellegrini, M. Morganti, V. Carnicelli, S. Cosio, O. Gagetti, A. R. Genazzani, and G. Bevilacqua. 1997. "p53 Alterations Are Predictive of Chemoresistance and Aggressiveness in Ovarian Carcinomas: A Molecular and Immunohistochemical Study." *British Journal of Cancer* 75 (2): 230–35. https://doi.org/10.1038/bjc.1997.38.

[118] Reles, Angela, Wen H. Wen, Conway Gee, Michael F. Press, Angela Reles, Annette Schmider, Uta Kilian, et al. 2001. "Correlation of p53 Mutations with Resistance to Platinum-Based Chemotherapy and Shortened Survival in Ovarian Cancer." *Clinical Cancer Research* 7 (10): 2984–97.

[119] Zhang, Yu, Lan Cao, Daniel Nguyen, and Hua Lu. 2016. "*TP53* Mutations in Epithelial Ovarian Cancer." *Translational Cancer Research*. https://doi.org/10.21037/tcr.2016.08.40.

[120] Silwal-Pandit, Laxmi, Anita Langerød, and Anne Lise Børresen-Dale. 2017. "*TP53* Mutations in Breast and Ovarian Cancer." *Cold Spring Harbor Perspectives in Medicine* 7 (1). https://doi.org/10.1101/cshperspect.a026252.

[121] Brennan, Joseph A., Jay O. Boyle, Wayne M. Koch, Steven N. Goodman, Ralph H. Hruban, Yolanda J. Eby, Marion J. Couch, Arlene A. Forastiere, and David Sidransky. 1995. "Association between Cigarette Smoking and Mutation of the p53 Gene in Squamous-Cell Carcinoma of the Head and Neck." *New England Journal of Medicine* 332 (11): 712–17. https://doi.org/10.1056/NEJM199503163321104.

[122] Temam, Stéphane, Antoine Flahault, Sophie Périé, Guy Monceaux, Florence Coulet, Patrice Callard, Jean François Bernaudin, Jean Lacau St Guily, and Pierre Fouret. 2000. "p53 Gene Status as a

Predictor of Tumor Response to Induction Chemotherapy of Patients with Locoregionally Advanced Squamous Cell Carcinomas of the Head and Neck." *Journal of Clinical Oncology* 18 (2): 385–94. https://doi.org/10.1200/jco.2000.18.2.385.

[123] Poeta, M. Luana, Judith Manola, Meredith A. Goldwasser, Arlene Forastiere, Nicole Benoit, Joseph A. Califano, John A. Ridge, et al. 2007. "*TP53* Mutations and Survival in Squamous-Cell Carcinoma of the Head and Neck." *New England Journal of Medicine* 357 (25): 2552–61. https://doi.org/10.1056/NEJMoa073770.

[124] Geisler, Stacy A., Andrew F. Olshan, Mark C. Weissler, Jainwen Cai, William K. Funkhouser, Joanna Smith, and Katie Vick. 2002. "p16 and p53 Protein Expression as Prognostic Indicators of Survival and Disease Recurrence from Head and Neck Cancer." *Clinical Cancer Research* 8 (11): 3445–53.

[125] Koch, Wayne M., Joseph A. Brennan, Marianna Zahurak, Steven N. Goodman, William H. Westra, Donna Schwab, George H. Yoo, Ding Jen Lee, Arlene A. Forastiere, and David Sidransky. 1996. "p53 Mutation and Locoregional Treatment Failure in Head and Neck Squamous Cell Carcinoma." *Journal of the National Cancer Institute* 88 (21): 1580–86. https://doi.org/10.1093/jnci/88.21.1580.

[126] Osman, Iman, Eric Sherman, Bhuvanesh Singh, Ennapadam Venkatraman, Michael Zelefsky, George Bosl, Howard Scher, et al. 2002. "Alteration of p53 Pathway in Squamous Cell Carcinoma of the Head and Neck: Impact on Treatment Outcome in Patients Treated with Larynx Preservation Intent." *Journal of Clinical Oncology* 20 (13): 2980–87. https://doi.org/10.1200/JCO. 2002.06.161.

[127] Lavertu, Pierre, David J. Adelstein, Jonathan Myles, and Michelle Secic. 2001. "p53 and Ki-67 as Outcome Predictors for Advanced Squamous Cell Cancers of the Head and Neck Treated With Chemoradiotherapy." *Laryngoscope* 111 (11): 1878–92. https://doi.org/10.1097/00005537-200111000-00002.

[128] Tandon, Sankalap, Catrin Tudur-Smith, Richard D. Riley, Mark T. Boyd, and Terence M. Jones. 2010. "A Systematic Review of p53 as a Prognostic Factor of Survival in Squamous Cell Carcinoma of the

Four Main Anatomical Subsites of the Head and Neck." *Cancer Epidemiology Biomarkers and Prevention.* https://doi.org/10.1158/1055-9965.EPI-09-0981.

[129] Russo, Antonio, Simona Corsale, Valentina Agnese, Marcella Macaluso, Sandra Cascio, Loredana Bruno, Eva Surmacz, et al. 2006. "TP53 Mutations and S-Phase Fraction but Not DNA-Ploidy Are Independent Prognostic Indicators in Laryngeal Squamous Cell Carcinoma." *Journal of Cellular Physiology* 206 (1): 181–88. https://doi.org/10.1002/jcp.20447.

[130] Vikhanskaya, Faina, Ming Kei Lee, Marco Mazzoletti, Massimo Broggini, and Kanaga Sabapathy. 2007. "Cancer-Derived p53 Mutants Suppress p53-Target Gene Expression - Potential Mechanism for Gain of Function of Mutant p53." *Nucleic Acids Research* 35 (6): 2093–2104. https://doi.org/10.1093/nar/gkm099.

[131] Blagosklonny, Mikhail V., Jeffrey Toretsky, Sean Bohen, and Len Neckers. 1996. "Mutant Conformation of p53 Translated in Vitro or in Vivo Requires Functional HSP90." *Proceedings of the National Academy of Sciences of the United States of America* 93 (16): 8379–83. https://doi.org/10.1073/pnas.93.16.8379.

[132] Whitesell, Luke, Patrick D. Sutphin, Elizabeth J. Pulcini, Jesse D. Martinez, and Paul H. Cook. 1998. "The Physical Association of Multiple Molecular Chaperone Proteins with Mutant p53 Is Altered by Geldanamycin, an Hsp90-Binding Agent." *Molecular and Cellular Biology* 18 (3): 1517–24. https://doi.org/10.1128/mcb.18.3.1517.

[133] Li, Dun, Natalia D. Marchenko, Ramona Schulz, Victoria Fischer, Talia Velasco-Hernandez, Flaminia Talos, and Ute M. Moll. 2011. "Functional Inactivation of Endogenous MDM2 and CHIP by HSP90 Causes Aberrant Stabilization of Mutant p53 in Human Cancer Cells." *Molecular Cancer Research* 9 (5): 577–88. https://doi.org/10.1158/1541-7786.MCR-10-0534.

[134] Wiech, Milena, Maciej B. Olszewski, Zuzanna Tracz-Gaszewska, Bartosz Wawrzynow, Maciej Zylicz, and Alicja Zylicz. 2012. "Molecular Mechanism of Mutant p53 Stabilization: The Role of

HSP70 and MDM2." *PLoS ONE* 7 (12). https://doi.org/10.1371/journal.pone.0051426.

[135] Ayrault, Olivier, Michael D. Godeny, Christopher Dillon, Frederique Zindy, Patrick Fitzgerald, Martine F. Roussel, and Helen M. Beere. 2009. "Inhibition of Hsp90 via 17-DMAG Induces Apoptosis in a p53-Dependent Manner to Prevent Medulloblastoma." *Proceedings of the National Academy of Sciences of the United States of America* 106 (40): 17037–42. https://doi.org/10.1073/pnas.0902880106.

[136] Alexandrova, Evguenia M., and Ute M. Moll. 2017. "Depleting Stabilized GOF Mutant p53 Proteins by Inhibiting Molecular Folding Chaperones: A New Promise in Cancer Therapy." *Cell Death and Differentiation.* https://doi.org/10.1038/cdd.2016.145.

[137] Schulz-Heddergott, Ramona, Nadine Stark, Shelley J. Edmunds, Jinyu Li, Lena Christin Conradi, Hanibal Bohnenberger, Fatih Ceteci, Florian R. Greten, Matthias Dobbelstein, and Ute M. Moll. 2018. "Therapeutic Ablation of Gain-of-Function Mutant p53 in Colorectal Cancer Inhibits Stat3-Mediated Tumor Growth and Invasion." *Cancer Cell* 34 (2): 298-314.e7. https://doi.org/10.1016/j.ccell.2018.07.004.

[138] NIH. U.S. National Library of Medicine. ClinicalTrials.gov. "*GANNET53: Ganetespib in metastatic, p53-mutant, platinum-resistant ovarian cancer.*" Available at https://clinicaltrials.gov/ct2/show/results/NCT02012192?term=hSP90+inhibitor&recrs=h&draw=2&rank=4. Last accessed 8.11.2020.

[139] Blagosklonny, Mikhail V., Shana Trostel, Ganesh Kayastha, Zoya N. Demidenko, Lyubomir T. Vassilev, Larisa Y. Romanova, Susan Bates, and Tito Fojo. 2005. "Depletion of Mutant p53 and Cytotoxicity of Histone Deacetylase Inhibitors." *Cancer Research* 65 (16): 7386–92. https://doi.org/10.1158/0008-5472.CAN-04-3433.

[140] Li, D., N. D. Marchenko, and U. M. Moll. 2011. "SAHA Shows Preferential Cytotoxicity in Mutant p53 Cancer Cells by Destabilizing Mutant p53 through Inhibition of the HDAC6-Hsp90 Chaperone Axis." *Cell Death and Differentiation* 18 (12): 1904–13. https://doi.org/10.1038/cdd.2011.71.

[141] NIH. U.S. National Library of Medicine. ClinicalTrials.gov. "*Panobinostat or Placebo with Bortezomib and Dexamethasone in Patients with Relapsed Multiple Myeloma (PANORAMA-1).*" Available at https://clinicaltrials.gov/ct2/show/results/NCT01023308?term=hdac6&draw=2&rank=8 Last accessed 8.11.20.

[142] Halasi, Marianna, Bulbul Pandit, and Andrei L. Gartel. 2014. "Proteasome Inhibitors Suppress the Protein Expression of Mutant p53." *Cell Cycle* 13 (20): 3202–6. https://doi.org/10.4161/15384101.2014.950132.

[143] An, Won G., Yutaka Chuman, Tito Fojo, and Mikhail V. Blagosklonny. 1998. "Inhibitors of Transcription, Proteasome Inhibitors, and DNA-Damaging Drugs Differentially Affect Feedback of p53 Degradation." *Experimental Cell Research* 244 (1): 54–60. https://doi.org/10.1006/excr.1998.4193.

[144] Choudhury, Sujata, Vamsi K. Kolukula, Anju Preet, Chris Albanese, and Maria Laura Avantaggiati. 2013. "Dissecting the Pathways That Destabilize Mutant p53: The Proteasome or Autophagy?" *Cell Cycle*. https://doi.org/10.4161/cc.24128.

[145] Yan, Wensheng, Yanhong Zhang, Jin Zhang, Shou Liu, Seong Jun Cho, and Xinbin Chen. 2011. "Mutant p53 Protein Is Targeted by Arsenic for Degradation and Plays a Role in Arsenic-Mediated Growth Suppression." *Journal of Biological Chemistry* 286 (20): 17478–86. https://doi.org/10.1074/jbc.M111.231639.

[146] Yan, Wensheng, Yong Sam Jung, Yanhong Zhang, and Xinbin Chen. 2014. "Arsenic Trioxide Reactivates Proteasome-Dependent Degradation of Mutant p53 Protein in Cancer Cells in Part via Enhanced Expression of Pirh2 E3 Ligase." *PLoS ONE* 9 (8). https://doi.org/10.1371/journal.pone.0103497.

[147] NIH. U.S. National Library of Medicine. ClinicalTrials.gov. *Arsenic Trioxide in Recurrent and Metastatic Ovarian Cancer and Endometrial Cancer With p53 Mutation.* Available at https://clinicaltrials.gov/ct2/show/NCT04489706?term=arsenic+trioxide&draw=2&rank=4. Last accessed 8/15/20.

[148] Wieczorek, Ania M., Jennifer L. F. Waterman, Matthew J. F. Waterman, and Thanos D. Halazonetis. 1996. "Structure-Based Rescue of Common Tumor-Derived p53 Mutants." *Nature Medicine* 2 (10): 1143–46. https://doi.org/10.1038/nm1096-1143.

[149] Brachmann, Rainer K., Kexin Yu, Yolanda Eby, Nikola P. Pavletich, and Jef D. Boeke. 1998. "Genetic Selection of Intragenic Suppressor Mutations That Reverse the Effect of Common p53 Cancer Mutations." *EMBO Journal* 17 (7): 1847–59. https://doi.org/10.1093/emboj/17.7.1847.

[150] Selivanova, Galina, Takashi Kawasaki, Ludmila Ryabchenko, and Klas G. Wiman. 1998. "Reactivation of Mutant p53: A New Strategy for Cancer Therapy." *Seminars in Cancer Biology* 8 (5): 369–78. https://doi.org/10.1006/scbi.1998.0099.

[151] Nikolova, Penka V., Kam Bo Wong, Brian DeDecker, Julia Henckel, and Alan R. Fersht. 2000. "Mechanism of Rescue of Common p53 Cancer Mutations by Second-Site Suppressor Mutations." *EMBO Journal* 19 (3): 370–78. https://doi.org/10. 1093/emboj/19.3.370.

[152] Selivanova, Galina, Violetta Iotsova, Ismail Okan, Michael Fritsche, Marika Ström, Bernd Groner, Roland C. Grafström, and Klas G. Wiman. 1997. "Restoration of the Growth Suppression Function of Mutant p53 by a Synthetic Peptide Derived from the p53 C-Terminal Domain." *Nature Medicine* 3 (6): 632–38. https://doi.org/10.1038/nm0697-632.

[153] Bykov, Vladimir J. N., Natalia Issaeva, Alexandre Shilov, Monica Hultcrantz, Elena Pugacheva, Peter Chumakov, Jan Bergman, Klas G. Wiman, and Galina Selivanova. 2002. "Restoration of the Tumor Suppressor Function to Mutant p53 by a Low-Molecular-Weight Compound." *Nature Medicine* 8 (3): 282–88. https://doi.org/10.1038/nm0302-282.

[154] Wiman, K. G. 2010. "Pharmacological Reactivation of Mutant p53: From Protein Structure to the Cancer Patient." *Oncogene*. https://doi.org/10.1038/onc.2010.188.

[155] Bykov, Vladimir J.N., Nicole Zache, Helene Stridh, Jacob Westman, Jan Bergman, Galina Selivanova, and Klas G. Wiman. 2005.

"PRIMA-1MET Synergizes with Cisplatin to Induce Tumor Cell Apoptosis." *Oncogene* 24 (21): 3484–91. https://doi.org/10.1038/sj.onc.1208419.

[156] Lehmann, Sören, Vladimir J. N. Bykov, Dina Ali, Ove Andreń, Honar Cherif, Ulf Tidefelt, Bertil Uggla, et al. 2012. "Targeting p53 in Vivo: A First-in-Human Study with p53-Targeting Compound APR-246 in Refractory Hematologic Malignancies and Prostate Cancer." *Journal of Clinical Oncology* 30 (29): 3633–39. https://doi.org/10.1200/JCO.2011.40.7783.

[157] Deneberg, S., H. Cherif, V. Lazarevic, P. O. Andersson, M. von Euler, G. Juliusson, and S. Lehmann. 2016. "An Open-Label Phase I Dose-Finding Study of APR-246 in Hematological Malignancies." *Blood Cancer Journal* 6 (7): e447. https://doi.org/10.1038/bcj.2016.60.

[158] NIH. U.S. National Library of Medicine. ClinicalTrials.gov. *p53 Suppressor Activation in Recurrent High Grade Serous Ovarian Cancer, a Phase Ib/II Study of Systemic Carboplatin Combination Chemotherapy With or Without APR-24.* Available at https://clinicaltrials.gov/ct2/show/NCT02098343?term=apr-246&draw=2&rank=8. Last accessed 8/8/2020.

[159] Cheok, Chit Fang, and David Philip Lane. 2017. "Exploiting the p53 Pathway for Therapy." *Cold Spring Harbor Perspectives in Medicine* 7 (3). https://doi.org/10.1101/cshperspect.a026310.

[160] Weissmueller, Susann, Eusebio Manchado, Michael Saborowski, John P. Morris IV, Elvin Wagenblast, Carrie A. Davis, Sung Hwan Moon, et al. 2014. "Mutant p53 Drives Pancreatic Cancer Metastasis through Cell-Autonomous PDGF Receptor β Signaling." *Cell* 157 (2): 382–94. https://doi.org/10.1016/j.cell.2014.01.066.

[161] Oden-Gangloff, A., F. Di Fiore, F. Bibeau, A. Lamy, G. Bougeard, F. Charbonnier, F. Blanchard, et al. 2009. "*TP53* Mutations Predict Disease Control in Metastatic Colorectal Cancer Treated with Cetuximab-Based Chemotherapy." *British Journal of Cancer* 100 (8): 1330–35. https://doi.org/10.1038/sj.bjc.6605008.

[162] Mounawar, Mounia, Anush Mukeria, Florence Le Calvez, Rayjean J. Hung, Helene Renard, Alexis Cortot, Claire Bollart, et al. 2007.

"Patterns of EGFR, HER2, *TP53*, and KRAS Mutations of P14arf Expression in Non-Small Cell Lung Cancers in Relation to Smoking History." *Cancer Research* 67 (12): 5667–72. https://doi.org/10.1158/0008-5472.CAN-06-4229.

[163] Sauer, L., D. Gitenay, C. Vo, and V. T. Baron. 2010. "Mutant p53 Initiates a Feedback Loop That Involves Egr-1/EGF Receptor/ERK in Prostate Cancer Cells." *Oncogene* 29 (18): 2628–37. https://doi.org/10.1038/onc.2010.24.

[164] Wang, W., B. Cheng, L. Miao, Y. Me, and M. Wu. 2013. "Mutant p53-R273H Gains New Function in Sustained Activation of EGFR Signaling via Suppressing MiR-27a Expression." *Cell Death and Disease* 4 (4). https://doi.org/10.1038/cddis.2013.97.

[165] Cheok, C. F., N. Kua, P. Kaldis, and D. P. Lane. 2010. "Combination of Nutlin-3 and VX-680 Selectively Targets p53 Mutant Cells with Reversible Effects on Cells Expressing Wild-Type p53." *Cell Death and Differentiation* 17 (9): 1486–1500. https://doi.org/10.1038/cdd.2010.18.

[166] Levesque, Aime A., Ethan A. Kohn, Edward Bresnick, and Alan Eastman. 2005. "Distinct Roles for p53 Transactivation and Repression in Preventing UCN-01-Mediated Abrogation of DNA Damage-Induced Arrest at S and G2 Cell Cycle Checkpoints." *Oncogene* 24 (23): 3786–96. https://doi.org/10.1038/sj.onc.1208451.

[167] Singh, Shilpa, Catherine A. Vaughan, Rebecca A. Frum, Steven R. Grossman, Sumitra Deb, and Swati Palit Deb. 2017. "Mutant p53 Establishes Targetable Tumor Dependency by Promoting Unscheduled Replication." *Journal of Clinical Investigation* 127 (5): 1839–55. https://doi.org/10.1172/JCI87724.

[168] Russell, Kenneth J., Denise A. Galloway, Sharon E. Plon, Mark Groudine, and Mark Groudine. 1995. "Abrogation of the G2 Checkpoint Results in Differential Radiosensitization of G1 Checkpoint-Deficient and G1 Checkpoint-Competent Cells." *Cancer Research* 55 (8): 1639–42.

[169] Wang, Qizhi, Saijun Fan, Alan Eastman, Peter J. Worland, Edward A. Sausville, and Patrick M. O'Connor. 1996. "UCN-01: A Potent

Abrogator of G2 Checkpoint Function in Cancer Cells with Disrupted p53." *Journal of the National Cancer Institute* 88 (14): 956–65. https://doi.org/10.1093/jnci/88.14.956.

[170] Nghiem, Paul, Peter K. Park, Yong Son Kim, Cyrus Vaziri, and Stuart L. Schreiber. 2001. "ATR Inhibition Selectively Sensitizes G1 Checkpoint-Deficient Cells to Lethal Premature Chromatin Condensation." *Proceedings of the National Academy of Sciences of the United States of America* 98 (16): 9092–97. https://doi.org/10.1073/pnas.161281798.

[171] Reaper, Philip M., Matthew R. Griffiths, Joanna M. Long, Jean Damien Charrier, Somhairle MacCormick, Peter A. Charlton, Julian M. C. Golec, and John R. Pollard. 2011. "Selective Killing of ATM- or p53-Deficient Cancer Cells through Inhibition of ATR." *Nature Chemical Biology* 7 (7): 428–30. https://doi.org/10.1038/nchembio.573.

[172] Vermeij, R, N Leffers, S. H. Van Der Burg, C J Melief, T Daemen, and H W Nijman. 2011. "Immunological and Clinical Effects of Vaccines Targeting p53-Overexpressing Malignancies." *Journal of Biomedicine and Biotechnology* 2011 (5015). https://doi.org/10.1155/2011/702146.

In: p53
Editor: Monte Stevens

ISBN: 978-1-53618-771-7
© 2020 Nova Science Publishers, Inc.

Chapter 3

p53-MEDIATED NEUROPROTECTIVE EFFECTS OF NATURAL COMPOUNDS IN OXIDATIVE STRESS CONDITIONS

*Klara Zubčić[1], Goran Šimić[1]
and Maja Jazvinšćak Jembrek[2,3]*

[1]Department for Neuroscience, Croatian Institute for Brain Research, University of Zagreb Medical School, Zagreb, Croatia
[2]Division of Molecular Medicine, Ruđer Bošković Institute, Zagreb, Croatia
[3]Department of Psychology, Catholic University of Croatia, Zagreb, Croatia

ABSTRACT

The transcription factor p53 orchestrates cellular response to different types of genotoxic challenges, including oxidative stress (OS). OS is induced by increased accumulation of reactive oxygen species and is tightly linked to the pathogenesis of various neurodegenerative diseases. During OS p53 undergoes posttranslational modifications that trigger its transcriptional activities, leading to activation of pro-apoptotic genes and repression of anti-apoptotic targets. In addition, p53 activity brings neurons into a more severe pro-oxidant condition based on the p53-driven activation of pro-oxidant genes and suppression of anti-oxidant genes. Recent studies suggest that dietary phytochemicals, such as flavonoids, may exert neuroprotective effects by downregulating expression of p53 gene *TP53* and acting along p53 pathways. In this chapter we will summarize recent findings related to the p53-mediated neuroprotective effects of natural compounds at the cellular, molecular, and behavioral level in various *in vitro* and *in vivo* models of neurodegenerative diseases, with a focus on Alzheimer's disease. Better understanding of the p53-mediated effects in neuroprotection may contribute to the development of more effective pharmacological approaches to OS-driven neurodegeneration.

ABBREVIATIONS

Aβ	amyloid β
AD	Alzheimer's disease
ALS	amyotrophic lateral sclerosis
APP	Aβ precursor protein
cdk5	cyclin-dependent kinase 5
EGCG	epigallocatechin-3-gallate
HD	Huntington's disease
HIPK2	homeodomain interacting protein kinase 2
HNE	4-hydroxy-2-nonenal
H_2O_2	hydrogen peroxide
HUVECs	human umbilical vein endothelial cells
GSH-Px	*glutathione peroxidase (E.C. 1.11.1.9)*
GSK-3β	*glycogen synthase kinase-3β (E.C. 2.7.11.26)*
MAPKs	mitogen-activated protein kinases
MDA	malondialdehyde
Mdm2	murine double minute-2
MNNG	*N*-methyl-*N'*-nitro-*N*-nitrosoguanidine
MPP$^+$	1-methyl-4-phenylpyridinium
mPTP	mitochondrial permeability transition pore
MPTP	1-methyl-4-phenyl-1,2,3,6-tetrahydropyridine

mtDNA	mitochondrial DNA
NMDA	*N*-methyl-D-aspartate
NOS	nitric oxide synthase
NOS2	inducible nictic oxide synthase gene
3-NP	3-nitropropionic acid
OS	oxidative stress
6-OHDA	6-hydroxydopamine
PD	Parkinson´s disease
PINK1	phosphatase and tensin homolog (PTEN)-induced kinase
PUMA	p53-upregulated mediator of apoptosis
ROS	reactive oxygen species
SIRT1	silent information regulator 1
SOD	superoxide dismutase
TIGAR	*TP53*-induced glycolysis and apoptosis regulator
TP53	p53 gene (tumor protein 53)

BIOLOGICAL FUNCTIONS AND STRUCTURE OF p53

Protein p53, also called "the guardian of the genome," is a redox-regulated transcription factor that controls cellular response to DNA damage. It maintains genome stability and is mostly known due to its ability to prevent tumor progression. p53 also modulates different metabolic functions, such as glycolysis, oxidative phosphorylation, synthesis and oxidation of fatty acids, among others (Liu et al., 2015; Hafner et al., 2019). Together with p63 and p73, another two members of the p53 family, p53 coordinates cell cycling, senescence, apoptosis, and differentiation (Eizenberg et al., 1996; Bourdon, 2007; Wei et al., 2012; Wang et al., 2014). Deregulation of its activity jeopardizes cellular homeostasis and results in many disorders, including neurodegenerative ones (Stanga et al., 2010; Szybińska and Leśniak, 2017; Jazvinšćak Jembrek et al., 2018a).

Several p53 protein isoforms have been characterized in humans, and there are several functional domains that must work together to ensure p53 activity. These include two transactivation (TA) domains at the N-terminus, the central DNA-binding domain, the oligomerization domain, and the non-structured C-terminal part (Sullivan et al., 2018). *TP53* gene possesses two promoters, P1 and P2. Full-length isoforms that contain both TA domains originate from the P1 promoter, whereas transcription from the P2 promoter generates N-terminally truncated isoforms (ΔN) without TA domains (Wei et al., 2012; Vieler and Sanyal, 2018). By using alternative promoters, alternative initiation of translation from two sites within the P1 promoter, and by alternative splicing, *TP53* gene give rise to four major isoforms: full-length p53 and three truncated forms Δ40p53, Δ133p53, and Δ160p53 lacking first 39, 132, and 159 amino acids, respectively, at the N-terminus (Khouri and Bourdon, 2011; Wei et al., 2012; Vieler and Sanyal, 2018). Δ40p53 isoforms retain the second TA domain (TA2), whereas Δ133p53 and Δ160p53 isoforms are short of both TA domains and also lack part of the DNA-binding region (Murray-Zmijewski et al., 2006; Pehar et al., 2014). Additional α, β and γ isoforms of full-length p53 and all truncated forms are formed through alternative splicing (Khoury and Bourdon, 2011; Pehar et al., 2014; Anbarasan and Bourdon, 2019). Functional consequences of this isoform abundance are barely elucidated, particularly in the nervous system. In general, it is known that only full-length p53 associates into the transcriptionally active tetrameric complex, whereas β and γ isoforms that lack oligomerization domain have reduced transcriptional activity (Wei et al., 2012; Anbarasan and Bourdon, 2019).

Various downstream targets of p53 are cellular mediators of its function. Isoforms of p63 and p73 with intact TA domain (TAp63 and TAp73) may also promote transcription of p53 target genes (Moll and Slade, 2004), while ΔN truncated isoforms antagonize p53 function (Marcel et al., 2012). As it will be explained bellow, from the perspective of neurodegenerative diseases, particularly interesting p53-regulated genes are those involved in apoptosis, such as Bax and p53-upregulated mediator of apoptosis (PUMA), and genes implicated in the maintenance of oxidative homeostasis (Liu and Xu, 2011).

REGULATION OF p53 ACTIVITY

p53 is intrinsically very unstable and is present intracellularly only in minute concentrations. Its stability is mainly regulated by protein-protein interactions and post-translational modifications, and to a lesser extent by conformational state (Stanga et al., 2010). Homeodomain-interacting protein kinase 2 (HIPK2) is one of the p53 activators that induces posttranslational modifications and confers to the conformational stability of p53. In regard to Alzheimer's disease (AD), soluble amyloid β (Aβ) is involved in a degradation of HIPK2 that consequently may affect p53 activity and neuronal response to DNA damaging injury (Lanni et al., 2010). In physiological conditions, p53 activity is antagonized by its negative regulators, of which the principal one is murine double minute-2 (Mdm2), an E3 ubiquitin ligase that labels p53 for proteosomal degradation (Wang et al., 2011). Another important regulator is Mdm4. In response to severe damage, Mdm4 promotes Mdm2-guided degradation and participates in posttranslational modifications of p53 by promoting HIPK2-mediated phosphorylation at Ser46, thus downregulating proteins with anti-apoptotic activity (Mancini et al., 2016).

Some posttranslational modifications that are introduced following DNA damage, such as acetylation, nitration and methylation, may disturb interactions between p53 and Mdm2, thus promoting its nuclear accumulation (Šimić et al., 2000a) and enhancement of transcriptional activity (Puca et al., 2009; Wu and Chiang, 2009; Yakovlev et al., 2010). Mathematical modelling predicted that acetylated p53 activates Bax and stimulates pro-apoptotic response under severe DNA damage, whereas the pro-survival role of phosphorylated forms prevails during slight injury (Fan et al., 2014).

Regarding conformational state, it is known that p53 tetramers are important for initiating apoptotic response, p53 dimers for growth arrest, whereas monomers and inactive forms are associated with cell growth (Fischer et al., 2016). Accordingly, various p53-binding partners may affect oligomerization of p53 and guide cellular response to harmful agents (van Dieck et al., 2009).

It is also critical that subtle changes in p53 activity may be achieved by redox status and zinc availability. Although reactive oxygen species (ROS) may activate p53, it is reported that oxidative conditions may inhibit binding of p53 to DNA by disrupting its conformation, thus conferring to the loss of p53 activity (Phatak and Muller, 2015). On the other hand, in reduced environment p53 binds zinc in the core domain and adopts conformation for DNA binding (Bykov et al., 2009).

p53 Effects during Neuronal Injury

p53 expression is upregulated in both acutely damaged neurons, and in the brain of patients with chronic neurodegenerative processes, clearly suggesting an important role of p53 in response to neuronal injury (Chang et al., 2012; Szybińska and Leśniak, 2017; Jazvinšćak Jembrek et al., 2018a).

Although p53 predominantly exerts its function by regulating expression of its pro-apoptotic downstream targets Bax and PUMA, in non-neuronal cells it may act by a transcription-independent mechanism. Direct interaction of p53 with the regulators of apoptosis from the Bcl-2 family may cause permeabilization of the outer mitochondrial membrane and induce apoptotic machinery (Schuler and Green, 2005; Speidel, 2010). In mature cortical neurons, the transcription-independent mode of action is likely not operative. Instead, apoptotic action of p53 in neuronal cells is mostly mediated by PUMA, a Bcl2-family member critically involved in neuronal death. PUMA initiates Bax-directed permeabilization of the outer mitochondrial membrane, which results in the release of the cytochromes c and activation of initiator and executioner caspases, thus triggering apoptosis (Steckley et al., 2007; Chatoo et al., 2011; Radovanović et al., 2019; Zubčić et al., 2020). However, translocation of p53 to mitochondria during OS has been demonstrated in human neuroblastoma cells SH-SY5Y, indicating that mitochondrial p53 activity could be involved in neuronal apoptosis, at least in some conditions (Park et al., 2015).

A part of p53 effects is mediated by sirtuins. p53 is important substrate of sirtuins, a class of proteins with deacetylase activity. In general, deacetylation of p53 decreases its transcriptional activity (Lee and Gu, 2013). p53 is acetylated in response to DNA damage, which results in its stabilization and induction of apoptosis. Consequently, increased p53 acetylation has been detected following exposure to various neurotoxic stimuli (Kim et al., 2007; Okawara et al., 2007). Similarly, histone deacetylase inhibitors protected neurons from several apoptotic insults by supressing p53-dependent expression of PUMA. This prevented activation of Bax and upregulation of caspase activity (Uo et al., 2009).

Besides regulating apoptotic events, p53 may be involved in necrotic death and autophagy. Generally, it is observed that in stress conditions p53 behaves as an autophagy-promoting factor as based on its transcriptional activity, whereas cytoplasmic p53 inhibits autophagy in physiological conditions through a transcription-independent mechanism (Park et al., 2016; Goiran et al., 2018). In one study, p53 was activated in mixed apoptotic and autophagic response following excitotoxic neuronal injury. Intrastriatal administration of quinolinic acid, an N-methyl-D-aspartate (NMDA) receptor agonist, upregulated p53 and increased expression of its pro-apoptotic and autophagic downstream targets (Wang et al. 2009). p53 also may regulate necrotic death after energetic collapse of the cell through the opening of the mitochondrial permeability transition pore (mPTP). Thus, p53 regulates OS-induced necrosis during brain ischemia/reperfusion injury. After accumulation in mitochondrial matrix, it triggers mPTP opening and initiates necrosis by physically interacting with cyclophilin D, a permeability transition pore regulator (Vaseva et al., 2012). Association of p53 with cyclophilin D is also required for the mPTP opening and apoptosis-independent death after oxygen-glucose deprivation/re-oxygenation induced neuronal death (Zhao et al., 2013a).

Many lines of evidence indicate that inhibition of p53-mediated apoptotic cascade may reduce neuronal damage and delay neuronal death. Lack of p53, or inhibition of its activity with the specific and reversible p53 inhibitor pifithrin-α, alleviates detrimental effects of various acute stressors (Morrison and Kinoshita, 2000; Culmsee et al., 2001; Plesnila et al., 2007), whereas overexpression of p53 induces widespread neuronal death (Jordán et al., 1997). Thus, pifithrin-α protects neurons against glutamate-, Aβ- and

DNA damaging agents-induced apoptosis in hippocampal and cortical cultures, as well as against hydrogen peroxide (H_2O_2)-induced OS in SH-SY5Y cells (Culmsee et al., 2001; Rachmany et al., 2013). In mice expressing two *p53* alleles (*p53*$^{+/+}$), as well as in mice heterozygous for *p53* (*p53*$^{+/-}$), extensive degeneration and loss of pyramidal neurons is observed in multiple brain regions (including hippocampus, amygdala, primary olfactory [piriform] cortex, cerebral cortex, and thalamus) following kainate injection, whereas *p53* knock-out mice are resistant (Morrison et al., 1996). As an inhibitor of transcriptional p53 activity, pifithrin-α reduces DNA-binding activity of p53. Consequently, it decreases production of Bax, a p53 target, diminishes mitochondrial dysfunction, and attenuates increase of caspase activity (Culmsee et al., 2001). Neuronal death after traumatic brain injury is also accompanied with a rapid p53 accumulation, its nuclear translocation, and decline in NF-κB transcriptional activity. In the presence of pifithrin-α, expression of NF-κB target proteins is upregulated together with reduced neurodegeneration, further indicating that the mechanism of p53-mediated death is dependent on the inhibition of NF-κB survival signaling (Plesnila et al., 2007). Similarly, in neuronal apoptosis provoked by kainic acid-induced seizures, p53 levels are increased (Sakhi et al., 1996), whereas seizure-induced hippocampal lesions, cognitive impairment, and neuronal death can be reduced by pharmacological inhibition of p53. Application of pifithrin-α also prevents induction of PUMA (Steckley et al., 2007; Engel et al., 2010; Rachmany et al., 2013). Furthermore, in mice administered with pifithrin-α, cortical and striatal neurons are more resistant to focal ischemic injury, whereas hippocampal neurons exhibit reduced excitotoxic damage (Culmsee et al., 2001). Likewise, pifithrin-α is effective against kainate-induced excitotoxicity in primary cortical cultures. It prevents neuronal death by preventing loss of mitochondrial membrane potential and dendrite degeneration (Neema et al., 2005). Pifithrin-α also protects striatal neurons after traumatic brain injury. It alleviates oxidative damage, apoptosis and autophagy, supresses glial activation, and improves motor deficits in rats (Huang et al., 2018).

Increase in p53 immunoreactivity is observed in cortical neurons and glial cells in brain areas affected by AD (Kitamura et al., 1997; Ohyagi et al., 2005). Astrocytes express two p53 isoforms, Δ133p53 and p53β, which differentially affect neuronal functioning. Isoform p53β is associated with the toxic effects of astrocytes on neuronal cells and its expression is upregulated in astrocytes of AD patients, while the expression of protective isoform Δ133p53 is depleted (Turnquist et al., 2016). Besides, increased expression of neuronal (constitutive) nitric oxide synthase (nNOS) is evident in reactive astrocytes surrounding Aβ plaques in the hippocampal formation and entorhinal cortex of AD patients. As neuronal DNA fragmentation is in a correlation with the localization of nNOS-expressing astrocytes, it has been suggested that upregulated generation of NO may be related to OS in AD (Šimić et al., 2000b). Furthermore, it has been found that p53 indirectly stimulates phosphorylation of tau protein, a major histopathological hallmark of AD (Hooper et al., 2007; Šimić et al., 2016), and also may interact with tau (Farmer et al., 2020). It has been shown that Δ40p53 isoform promotes tau phosphorylation via transcriptional activation of several tau kinases, and its level increases during aging (Phar et al., 2014). Increase in p53 expression in AD is affected by the accumulation of Aβ. Aβ42 directly activates *TP53* promoter, and OS induces nuclear localization of Aβ42, thus increasing p53 expression (Ohyagi et al., 2005).

It has been also demonstrated that levels of p53 monomers and dimers are elevated in AD brains, and that these forms of p53 are selectively glutathionylated. Therefore, it has been hypothesized that glutathionylation prevents formation of active tetrameric forms that potentially might have some implications for the pathogenesis of AD (Di Domenico et al., 2009). Recently, it has been shown that phosphorylated p53 forms oligomers and fibrils in human AD brain. This phosphorylated p53 forms are mislocalized outside the nucleus, very likely underlying observed impairment of DNA damage response in AD (Farmer et al., 2020). Besides, p53 regulates expression of some microRNAs (miRNAs), including members of the miR-34 family, which are implicated in various brain disorders (Rokavec et al., 2014).

On the other hand, in addition to detrimental outcomes after transcriptional activation of p53, several studies have demonstrated protective potential of p53. In a *Drosophila* model of tau pathology, p53 exerts beneficial effects by controlling expression of genes important for synaptic functioning (Merlo et al., 2014). Furthermore, acetylated p53 is needed for neurite outgrowth in primary neuronal cultures and axonal regeneration in mice models, where it transactivates promoters of actin-binding protein Coronin 1b and the GTPase Rab13 that interact with the cytoskeleton network (Di Giovanni et al., 2006; Di Giovanni and Rathore, 2012).

OXIDATIVE STRESS

OS is one of the major causes of cellular damage in neurodegeneration. OS denotes condition in which various endogenous mechanisms of enzymatic and non-enzymatic antioxidative defence are overwhelmed by an increased production of reactive oxygen and nitrogen species (ROS and RNS, respectively). In the pathogenesis of AD, OS is considered as an early event that precedes the onset of clinical symptoms (Multhaup et al., 2002; Šimić et al., 2009; Bonda et al., 2010). Ultimately, ROS an RNS, as highly reactive species, cause damage to all biological macromolecules (including DNA, which represents the major trigger for p53 activation), deregulate mitochondrial function and ATP production further facilitating cumulative damage by free radicals, induce endoplasmic reticulum stress response, impair synaptic function, disturb elimination of damaged proteins and organelles by the proteosomal system and autophagy, and initiate widespread microglial activation and consequent neuronal inflammation pathways (Šimić et al., 2019; Španić et al., 2019). All these events result in neuronal death and appearance of behavioral, emotional, and cognitive changes that are specific for each neurodegenerative disorder (Bonda et al., 2010; Kim et al., 2015; Liu et al., 2017; Jazvinšćak Jembrek et al., 2015;2018a).

Dysregulation of metal homeostasis is one of the most important factors that contributes to OS generation in neurodegeneration. Transient metals such as copper and zinc are particularly relevant in this context. They catalyse production of ROS in a Fenton-type reaction, thus promoting OS conditions and neuronal damage (Multhaup et al., 2002; Jazvinšćak Jembrek et al., 2014; Radovanović et al., 2019; Zubčić et al., 2020). In AD, Aβ aggregates bind transition metal ions and promote production of ROS via redox cycling (Phatak and Muller, 2015; Cheignon et al., 2018). Aβ is also accumulated in mitochondrial matrix, where it modulates protein turnover. This further contributes to mitochondrial failure and dysregulation of ROS production (Chen and Yan, 2007; Mossmann et al., 2017; Cheignon et al., 2018). In addition, OS is tightly involved in tau hyperphosphorylation. Tau is a microtubule-associated protein with the important role in the maintenance of microtubule stability. When tau is hyperphosphorylated, its affinity for microtubules is reduced, which destabilizes cytoskeletal architecture, axonal transport, and overall neuronal functioning (Šimić et al., 2016; Guo et al., 2017). Prolonged OS activates many kinases involved in tau phosphorylation, including *glycogen synthase kinase-3β (GSK-3β, Jazvinšćak Jembrek et al., 2013)*, cyclin-dependent kinase 5 (cdk5) and mitogen-activated protein kinases (MAPKs) JNK and p38, and supresses activity of tau-related phosphatases, of which the most important is protein phosphatase 2A (PP2A), ultimately leading to the hyperphosphorylation of tau and impairment of its function (Su et al., 2010; Alavi Naini and Soussi-Yanicostas, 2015; Šimić et al., 2016). p53 also indirectly contributes to tau phosphorylation (Hooper et al., 2007).

p53 AND OXIDATIVE STRESS

Intracellular production of ROS is partially determined by p53. In physiological conditions, p53 participates in maintaining basal levels of ROS by controlling transcription of antioxidative enzymes such as glutathione-peroxidase (GSH-Px) and repressing pro-oxidative genes, such as inducible nitric oxide synthase (*NOS2*). As a net result of these activities, in healthy neurons p53 predominantly functions as a pro-oxidant, although it does not have to be necessarily considered harmful.

It has been hypothesized that overall pro-oxidative activity of p53 might have some unrecognized, beneficial role in synaptic functioning or neuronal plasticity (Chatoo et al., 2011). Accordingly, loss of p53 activity reduces the overall physiological level of OS in mice brain (Barone et al., 2012). In p53 knock-out mouse, the basal OS is reduced as mirrored by decreased protein carbonyl content and reduced amount of protein-bound 4-hydroxy-2-nonenal (HNE), an end product of lipid peroxidation, in comparison with wild-type animals. These changes are accompanied with the reduced levels of transcription factor Nrf2 and upregulation of NF-κB, thioredoxin-1, and superoxide dismutase 2 (SOD2) (Barone et al., 2012). Hence, pharmacological approach directed toward the attenuation of p53 and its pro-oxidative action could be a promising approach in slowing down progression of OS-mediated neurodegenerative changes.

In regard to OS, the threshold for p53 activation is lower in neurons than in other tissues (Chatoo et al., 2011). It is interesting that p53-mediated response to oxidative injury is guided by the severity of the cellular damage. When the environment is mildly oxidative, p53 contributes to cell survival by activating transcription of anti-oxidative genes. On the contrary, if cellular functioning is seriously jeopardized, p53-mediated transcription is switched to a pro-oxidative mode, and p53 activity results in creating more severe pro-oxidative environment, leading to cell death (Liu and Xu, 2011). p53 stimulates production of ROS via at least two mechanisms. First, it stimulates transcription of pro-oxidative, ROS-generating enzymes, as well as pro-apoptotic proteins that disturb electron transport chain in mitochondria (including Bax and PUMA). Second, it supresses transcription of anti-oxidative genes, such as mitochondrial manganese-containing SOD, i.e., *SOD2* (Culmsee and Mattson, 2005; Liu et al. 2008; Holley et al., 2010). Yet another p53-inducible gene is *TIGAR* (TP53-induced glycolysis and apoptosis regulator), which inhibits glycolysis and thus reduces overall ROS production. Hence, p53 expression offers protection against oxidative damage and ROS-initiated apoptosis in AD (Katsel et al., 2013).

p53 AND MITOCHONDRIAL FUNCTION

Mitochondria-related p53 functions attracted growing interest when considering OS, neuronal aging, and neurodegeneration. OS, as an early event in the course of neurodegeneration, may be triggered by the impairment of mitochondrial function, and vice versa, mitochondrial damage can be induced by the increased OS. Furthermore, dysregulated production of ROS may induce mutations in mitochondrial DNA, disturb respiratory chain, membrane potential and permeability, and disrupt Ca^{2+} homeostasis further compromising mitochondrial functions (Guo et al., 2013a). In cellular models of AD, even subtoxic, 1 µM concentrations of $A\beta_{1-42}$, are sufficient to elicit dramatic changes in mitochondrial health, as revealed by an increase of oxidative adducts, up-regulation of the full-length mitochondrial DNA (mtDNA), and extensive fragmentation of the unamplified mtDNA (Diana et al., 2008).

From what we know today, p53 controls mitochondria at many levels. At first, p53 regulates mitophagy, a specific autophagy-based process for the selective degradation of damaged, ROS-producing mitochondria. It has been shown that cytosolic p53 disables removal of damaged mitochondria. p53 binds to protein Parkin and disturbs its translocation to mitochondria and activation of Parkin's E3 ubiquitin ligase, ultimately facilitating mitochondrial dysfunction (Hoshino et al., 2013; Zhang et al., 2020). Nuclear p53 activity also may down-regulate autophagy as p53 represses expression of phosphatase and tensin homolog (PTEN)-induced kinase 1 (PINK1), a pro-autophagic effector critically involved in the control of mitophagy (Goiran et al., 2018). Furthermore, many mitochondrial proteins participating in respiration and mitochondrial metabolism are regulated by p53, and their transcription may affect ROS production and mitochondrial function (Liu et al., 2008; Lacroix et al., 2020). p53 also helps in maintaining mitochondrial genome stability and integrity via its nuclear activity and by interacting with mitochondrial DNA repair proteins in mitochondria (Park et al., 2016). In addition, many mitochondrial fusion/fission proteins are regulated by p53. Maintenance of adequate number and shape of mitochondria is important for the fulfilment of high energy demands of neuronal cells. Optimal mitochondrial shape and size are not required only for energetic functioning, but also for proper mitochondrial transport along axons. Hence, mitochondrial dynamics is often compromised in neurodegeneration due to enhanced p53 expression (Wang et al., 2014). Finally, ample data have been accumulated that p53 is an important metabolic regulator, although the mechanisms underlying these p53 activities are only partly understood. It is known that p53 regulates cellular metabolism by promoting assembly of ATP synthase, glucose levels, and ATP production in glycolysis, as well as oxidative phosphorylation and glutamine and lipid metabolism (Liang et al. 2013; Lacroix et al. 2020). Although these non-transcriptional activities of p53 are not well understood in neuronal cells, they indicate that a plethora of cellular events at the mitochondrial level may be guided by p53, and that their regulation may represent pharmacological targets in neurodegeneration (for review, see Wang et al., 2014; Dai et al., 2016).

NATURAL COMPOUND AS MODULATORS OF p53 SIGNALING

Due to the important role of p53 in programmed cell death pathways, it is believed that p53-inhibiting agents could be beneficial against pathological events associated with neurodegenerative diseases (Culmsee and Mattson, 2005; Chang et al., 2012). In that sense, it is assumed that natural compounds capable of inhibiting p53 pathway might be useful in preventing and slowing down progression of neurodegenerative changes (Nakanishi et al., 2015). Besides modulating p53 signaling, phytochemicals may modulate other signaling cascades, act as antioxidants (by scavenging ROS, chelating excess of metal ions, and modulating expression of enzymatic and non-enzymatic antioxidative defence components), exhibit anti-apoptotic and other pro-survival activities, and restore mitochondrial functions, among others. Furthermore, they promote cerebrovascular blood flow and supress neuroinflammation and gliosis, altogether demonstrating a positive effect on cognitive functioning (Vauzour et al., 2008; Davinelli et al., 2016).

Indeed, many studies have demonstrated that phytochemicals capable of modulating p53 signaling may exert neuroprotective and health-promoting effects. Flavonoids, major polyphenolic products of secondary plant metabolism, are highly diverse and one of the most investigated group of dietary phytochemicals with the potential to act as preventive or therapeutic agents in neurodegenerative diseases (Ayaz et al., 2019; Maher, 2019; Maan et al., 2020). In their chemical structure there are two benzene rings (rings A and B) bridged with a pyran ring (ring C). Flavonoids are classified depending on the position at which B ring is attached to C ring, the degree of oxidation and unsaturation of the central ring, the pattern of hydroxylation, and attached glycosidic moieties and other substituents. Major groups of flavonoids are flavonols, flavanols, flavones, flavanones, anthocyanins, and isoflavones (Ayaz et al., 2019; Maher, 2019).

Quercetin from the flavonol group is one of the most abundant flavonoids and one of the most potent scavengers of ROS with demonstrated neuroprotective properties (Jazvinšćak Jembrek et al., 2012a,b; Costa et al., 2016). Quercetin may directly interact with p53. It has been shown that quercetin binds to the ribonucleoside binding domain of p53 via several hydrogen bonds and one hydrophobic interaction (Amanzadeh et al., 2019). Quercetin protects rat pheochromocytoma (PC12) cells against H_2O_2-induced OS by reducing levels of ROS and malondialdehyde (MDA), an end product of lipid peroxidation. Furthermore, in these cells quercetin strongly upregulates antioxidative enzymes catalase, SOD and GSH-Px, restores Bcl-2/Bax ratio, and reduces caspase-3 cleavage and p53 expression, altogether preventing ROS-initiated neuronal apoptosis (Bao et al., 2017). Similarly, quercetin improves survival of H_2O_2-treated P19 neurons by alleviating p53 increase and downregulation of Bcl-2, and by modulating Akt and ERK1/2 signaling pathways (Jazvinšćak Jembrek et al., 2018b). Anti-oxidative and anti-apoptotic mechanisms of quercetin action have been also observed in P19 neurons exposed to copper-induced OS, although the levels of p53 protein were not affected by exposure to neither copper nor quercetin (Zubčić et al., 2020). Furthermore, quercetin may inhibit tau-fibril formation, probably by conformationally stabilizing tau monomers upon binding (Kumar et al., 2019). Quercetin also prevents okadaic acid-induced hyperphosphorylation of tau in HT22 hippocampal cells by inhibiting Ca^{2+}-calpain-p25-cdk5 pathway (Shen et al., 2018). In *Drosophila* AD model quercetin restores Aβ-induced changes in gene expression, including genes involved in OS response and p53 pathway (Kong et al., 2016), whereas in a 3xTg-AD mice preventive administration of quercetin for 12 months significantly reduces β-amyloid aggregation and partially prevents increase in hyperphosphorylated tau in the CA1 region of the hippocampus and amygdala with positive effects on cognitive performance (Paula et al., 2019). Solid lipid nanoparticles loaded with quercetin improve pentylenetetrazol-induced memory impairment in zebrafish together with restoring acetylcholinesterase activity, basal level of lipid peroxidation and glutathione content in the zebrafish brain, further demonstrating its neuroprotective potential (Rishitha and Muthuraman, 2018). In aluminium-induced neurodegeneration in the rat hippocampus quercetin reduced OS by decreasing ROS production and increasing mitochondrial SOD, and also downregulates p53, Bax and caspase-3 activation, and preserves mitochondrial morphology (Sharma et al., 2016). Quercetin also demonstrates neuroprotective effects in the rotenone rat model of Parkinson´s disease (PD). It attenuates rotenone-induced behavioral changes, but also stimulates autophagy, restores dopamine level and OS markers, and prevents neuronal necrosis (El-Horany et al., 2016). As rotenone treatment promotes p53 expression (Feng et al., 2015), and other flavonoids have been shown to attenuate rotenone-induced toxicity by supressing p53 expression (Li et al., 2011), it is possible that effects of quercetin against rotenone-induced toxicity are also mediated along p53 pathway. In 3-nitropropionic acid (3-NP)-induced model of Huntington's disease (HD), quercetin significantly improves mitochondrial dysfunctions, restores ATP levels, reduces mitochondrial OS, and preserves activities of SOD and catalase, together with ameliorating neurobehavioral deficits (Sandhir and Mehrotra, 2013). As all these parameters are p53-regulated, it is likely that effects of quercetin in this HD model are also achieved via p53 signaling. In conclusion, based on the observed neuroprotective effects of quercetin, both *in vitro* and in animal models, quercetin is highly appreciated for potential clinical applications, particularly in AD (Khan et al., 2019a).

Some other flavonoids from the class of flavonols also modulate p53 pathway and exhibit neuroprotective effects against OS-induced neurodegeneration. For example, rutin (vitamin P) protects rat brain against oxidative damage induced by transient focal ischemia. It reduces p53 expression and increases activity of endogenous mechanisms of antioxidative defence (Khan et al., 2009). In another model of oxidative injury, rutin prevents cognitive impairments and neuroinflammation (Javed et al., 2012), and is also capable to promote microglial Aβ clearance (Pan et al., 2019). Rutin treatment also restores colicistin-induced OS and apoptosis in male rats. Colicistin is an antibiotic that may induce axonal and neuronal damage. Among other effects, rutin restores brain function by attenuating colicistin-induced expression of OS and inflammation markers, and by supressing p53, ERK1/2 and caspase-3 activity that ultimately reduce number of apoptotic and necrotic neurons in rat hippocampus (Çelik et al., 2020). Yet another flavonol, fisetin, inhibits sumoylation of p53 and negatively affects biological activity of p53 (Velazhahan et al., 2020).

Catechins from the flavanol group, such as epigallocatechin-3-gallate (EGCG), the major polyphenolic compound from the green tea, are also widely studied. Many results indicate that they can be useful in the prevention and therapy of neurodegenerative pathologies (Singh et al., 2016; Pervin et al., 2018). Polyphenols from the green tea are powerful ROS scavengers and metal chelators capable to prevent lipid peroxidation and DNA damage, reduce caspase activity, and promote neuronal survival (Ayaz et al., 2019). Furthermore, EGCG may reduce soluble and insoluble forms of Aβ and sarkosyl-soluble phosphorylated tau isoforms in APPsw mice, and improve cognitive abilities (Rezai-Zadeh et al., 2008; Wobst et al., 2015). In cerebellar granule neurons, EGCG is particularly effective against mitochondrial OS as it probably accumulates in mitochondria and locally acts as ROS scavenger (Schroeder et al., 2009). In neuronal-like PC12 cells, EGCG inhibits NO-induced apoptosis by scavenging free radicals and preventing cytochrome c release and caspase-3 activation (Jung et al., 2007). EGCG also protects PC12 cells against copper-induced generation of ROS, and inhibited fibrillation of α-synuclein (a typical feature of PD) by forming Cu/EGCG complex that prevents transition of α-synuclein from random coil to β-sheet structure (Teng et al., 2019). In SH-SY5Y cells treated with 6-hydroxydopamine (6-OHDA), a neurotoxin that induces pathological changes characteristic for PD, EGCG restores activity of protein kinase C (PKC) and ERK1/2, and prevents 6-OHDA-induced increase in Bax and Mdm2. As Mdm2 is the major negative regulator of p53 that is often increased simultaneously with p53, the authors have hypothesized that EGCG likely regulates p53 levels (Levites et al., 2002). Besides, cancer research studies have demonstrated that EGCG may modulate p53-regulated apoptosis (Qin et al., 2008; Yamauchi et al., 2009).

Flavonoids from the flavanone subgroup also act as neuroprotective agents. Pre-treatment with naringin, a flavanone glycoside abundantly present in citrus fruit and capable of crossing blood-brain barrier, attenuates cytochrome c release and antiapoptotic effects in PC12 cells. In lipopolysaccharide-induced apoptosis that is associated with increased production of ROS and pro-inflammatory mediators, naringin improves viability, prevents ROS release and down-regulates pro-inflammatory genes, stimulates transcription of several antioxidative enzymes, decreases phosphorylation of MAPKs, and reduces expression of apoptosis-related genes, including *TP53*. In cells exposed only to lipopolysaccharide, p53 is critical inhibitor of antiapoptotic protein Bcl-2. The interaction between p53 and Bcl-2 promotes mitochondrial permeabilization and further initiation of apoptotic events (Wang et al., 2017). Naringin also protects PC12 cells from 3-NP-induced neurotoxicity by various mechanisms that could be p53-regulated. Thus, it increases activity of antioxidative enzymes, decreases ROS levels and lipid peroxidation, improves Bcl-2/Bax ratio and stimulates Akt signaling pathway (Kulasekaran and Ganapasam, 2015).

Apigenin and luteolin are flavonoids from the flavone subclass. They are both effective against oxidative injury and capable to modulate p53 pathway. For example, apigenin protects differentiated PC12 cells against OS and apoptosis induced by oxygen and glucose deprivation/reperfusion. It also affects mitochondrial membrane potential, levels of antioxidative and detoxifying enzymes, and expression of p53 and Nrf2 and their target genes

(Guo et al., 2014). Furthermore, apigenin prevents kainic acid-induced seizures and protects hippocampal neurons against excitotoxicity by attenuating ROS increase and glutathione depletion (Han et al., 2012), and protects cells against Aβ-mediated toxicity in the presence of copper by preserving redox balance and mitochondrial function, and by preventing ROS-mediated activation of p38 and JNK signaling and apoptosis (Zhao et al., 2013b). Like apigenin, luteolin may achieve neuroprotective effects via several different mechanisms, including ROS scavenging, induction of antioxidative enzymes, alleviation of mitochondrial injury, attenuation of inflammation and apoptosis, and stimulation of autophagy, all processes that are, at least in part, very likely regulated by p53 (Ashaari et al., 2018; Fu et al. 2018; Tan et al., 2020a). Luteolin also attenuates 6-OHDA-induced death of PC12 by downregulating p53, PUMA and Bax expression (Guo et al., 2013b; Hu et al., 2014), prevents apoptotic effects of Aβ in cultured cortical neurons by modulating caspase-3 activity and signaling via MAPK pathways (Cheng et al., 2010), and decreases zinc-induced tau hyperphosphorylation in SH-SY5Y cells through the attenuation of ROS production and activation of Akt and ERK1/2 pathways (Zhou et al., 2011; 2012). Several studies have demonstrated that its neuroprotective effects are related to Nrf2 transcriptional activity and decreased OS, including in the study performed in striatal cells obtained from the HD knock-in mice expressing mutant huntingtin protein (Oliveira et al., 2015; Tan et al., 2020a). Of note, interaction between Nrf2 and p53 has been demonstrated in luteolin-treated cancer cells too. Furthermore, it is known that p21, a p53 target, stabilizes Nrf2, whereas quinine oxidoreductase 1 (NQO1), an Nrf2 target, inhibits degradation of p53 (Kang et al., 2019). Luteolin also prevents methamphetamine-induced apoptosis and autophagy in rat striatum by modulating Akt pathway, and p53 and Bax expression (Tan et al., 2020b). Chrysin, yet another flavone, also exhibited neuroprotective effect by modulating p53 pathway. Its protection of SH-SY5Y cells against diclofenac-induced OS and apoptosis was associated with the attenuation of diclofenac-induced p53 increase (Darendelioglu, 2020).

Anthocyanins are class of flavonoids abundant in many vegetables, fruits, nuts and seed, particularly in berry fruits and red wine. Extracts enriched in anthocyanins and proanthocyanidins are effective against rotenone-induced OS and neuronal death of primary midbrain cultures (Strathearn et al., 2014). In SH-SY5Y dopaminergic cells, proanthocyanidins reverse rotenone-induced effects on cell survival, inhibit ROS generation and apoptosis-related changes such as caspase-3 activity and poly (ADP ribose) polymerase (PARP) cleavage, and attenuate signaling along p38, JNK and ERK pathways (Ma et al., 2018b). Proanthocyanidins from lotus seedpod ameliorate D-galactose-induced cognitive impairment, and reduce OS markers, Aβ levels, and p53 expression in the hippocampus of senescent mice (Gong et al., 2016). Suppression of p53 expression has been also recently demonstrated in other models of injury. Cinnamon procyanidin oligomers were shown to protect mice neurons against 1-methyl-4-phenyl-1,2,3,6-tetrahydropyridine (MPTP)-induced toxicity by regulating p38/p53/Bax pathway (Xu et al., 2020). Grape seed proanthocyanidin extract reduces thaliodomide- and carboplatin-induced brain damage, OS, and p53 increase, among other effects (Yousef et al., 2018). Similarly, anthocyanins are effective against focal cerebral ischemic injury in rats by suppressing upregulation of p53 and activation of JNK signaling (Shin et al., 2006). Treatment with various berry extracts rich in anthocyanins prevented ROS increase, activation of microglia, Aβ fibrillation, and apoptotic cascade *in vitro* (Ma et al., 2018a). In lipopolysaccharide-induced injury, anthocyanins reversed JNK activation and stimulate Akt signaling, reduce levels of inflammatory markers, attenuate apoptotic cascade and expression of Bax, a p53 target, and increase levels of synaptic proteins, thus improving hippocampus-dependent memory functions in treated mice (Khan et al., 2019b). Black chokeberry anthocyanins are protective against aging-related pathological changes when applied for eight weeks in mice. It seems that they help in the preservation of redox homeostasis, but also enhance monoamine levels, reduce levels of pro-inflammatory cytokines and expression of p53 and p-p53, which ultimately promote cognitive functioning in old mice (Wei et al., 2017).

Isoflavones are class of flavonoids naturally found in soy and soy products. Their molecular structure resembles estrogens (phytoestrogens).

Hence, they are mostly known due to their estrogen-like effects and alleviation of postmenopausal symptoms in women. However, they also have antiinflammatory and neuroprotective effects (Yu et al., 2019). When applied together with folic acid, soybean isoflavone prevents neural tube defects induced by cyclophosphamide. Moreover, this combination prevents apoptotic changes, lipid peroxidation, DNA damage, and p53 and Bax expression in embryonic rodent brains (Zhao et al., 2010). Genistein is one of the most studied isoflavone with promising potential against AD pathological changes due to its numerous beneficial effects. It possesses strong free radical scavenging capacity, upregulates antioxidant enzymatic activity, reduces OS, interferes with intracellular signaling – stimulates PI3K/Akt and Nrf2 pathways, downregulates neuroinflammation, inhibits apoptosis, decreases Aβ generation and prevents Aβ aggregation, activates Aβ-clearance pathway, reduces Aβ-induced neurotoxicity and Aβ-mediated activation of p38 MAPK (Uddin and Kabir, 2019). In Aβ$_{31-35}$ treated cultured cortical neurons genistein downregulates expression of p53 and Bax, as well as caspase-3 activity, thus preventing neuronal apoptosis (Yu et al., 2009). Puerarin (daidzein-8-C-glucoside), a major flavonoid from the *Pueraria lobata*, is another isoflavone with neuroprotective effects. Puerarin has shown to be effective against 1-methyl-4-phenylpyridinium (MPP$^+$)-induced death of SH-SY5Y cells. It upregulates Akt activity and prevents nuclear translocation of p53, as well as PUMA and Bax upregulation, and caspase-3 activity. Beneficial effect of puerarin can be abrogated by pifithrin-α, indicating critical role of p53 in its beneficial effects (Zhu et al., 2012).

Apart from flavonoids, some other compounds of natural origin are considered as possible protective agents against OS-induced neurodegeneration. Resveratrol is natural non-flavonoid polyphenolic compound abundantly present in red wine and skin of purple grapes that exerts antioxidant, anti-inflammatory, and neuroprotective effects. Resveratrol promotes Aβ clearance and expression of antioxidative enzymes, reduces toxicity and aggregation of Aβ, preserves energetic homeostasis, promotes neurogenesis but supresses microglial activation, and prevents apoptosis (Bastianetto et al., 2015; Gomes et al., 2018). In Aβtreated PC12 cells resveratrol prevents apoptotic death by decreasing Bax expression and caspase-3 activity, along with increasing p53 acetylation (Ai et al., 2015). In 3xTg-AD mice, two-month supplementation with resveratrol has been shown to prevent cognitive impairment and development of Aβ and tau pathology in the hippocampus. These effects have been accompanied with increased levels of protease neprilysin, depleted β secretase 1 (β-site APP cleavage enzyme, BACE1) levels, and have also enhanced ubiquitin-proteasome activity, along with depleted levels of acetylated p53 (Corpas et al., 2018). It is known that through AMP kinase induction resveratrol activates NAD^+-dependent deacetylase silent information regulator 1 (SIRT1) that consequently reduces levels of acetylated p53. Similarly, neuroprotective effects of resveratrol against rotenone-induced injury in SH-SY5Y cells are mediated via SIRT1 induction and decreased expression of total and acetylated p53 and reduced *TP53* gene expression, thus preventing p53-mediated apoptosis (Feng et al., 2015). Likewise, resveratrol protects PC12 cells against Aβ-induced apoptosis by upregulating SIRT1 (Feng et al. 2013). In yet another study, resveratrol treatment has prevented hippocampal neurodegeneration in the inducible p25 transgenic mice, a model of AD and other tauopathies that overexpresses cdk5 coactivator, by upregulating SIRT1 and decreasing p53 acetylation (Kim et al., 2007). Neuroprotection against NMDA-induced toxicity in cultured cortical neurons has been also achieved via upregulated SIRT1 and reduced levels of acetylated p53 (Yang et al., 2017). Induction of SIRT1 and beneficial role of resveratrol in neuroprotection has been observed in transgenic mice expressing mutant SOD1, a model of amyotrophic lateral sclerosis (ALS), in neurons treated with H_2O_2 (Kim et al., 2007), in organotypic midbrain slice culture exposed to dopaminergic neurotoxin MPP^+ (Okawara et al., 2007), and in a model of cerebral ischemia (oxygen glucose deprivation) in the organotypic hippocampal slice culture (Raval et al., 2006). Furthermore, treatment of dopaminergic neurons from midbrain slice cultures with *N*-methyl-*N'*-nitro-*N*-nitrosoguanidine (MNNG), a DNA alkylating agent, reduces p53 acetylation, probably due to deacetylating activity of sirtuins (Okawara et al., 2007). Neuroprotective effect of resveratrol against high glucose-induced OS in dopaminergic PC12 cells is also associated with reduced p53 expression in the nucleus and reduced expression of GRP75, a p53 inhibitor, in the cytoplasm (Renaud et al., 2014).

Thymoquinone is a bioactive compound from a widely used medicinal plant *Nigella sativa Linn*. It protects SH-SY5Y cells against H_2O_2-induced neurotoxicity. Thymoquinone restores activity of mitochondrial metabolic enzymes and attenuates H_2O_2-induced increase in ROS production. It upregulates expression of antioxidative enzymes SOD1, SOD2 and catalase, promotes expression of Akt1, ERK1/2, p38, JNK and NF-κB, but supresses expression of p53 mRNA (Ismail et al., 2018). In PC12 cells treated with $A\beta_{25-35}$ fragment, antioxidative properties of thymoquinone are also evident, further supporting its potential for AD treatment. Thymoquinone prevents noxious effects of Aβ on lipid peroxidation and NO production, and restores levels of glutathione, GSH-Px, and glutathione reductase (Khan et al., 2012). In line with these findings, in cultured hippocampal and cortical neurons treated with $A\beta_{1-42}$, thymoquinone also improves survival, inhibits collapse of mitochondrial membrane potential and increase in intracellular ROS levels, restores recycling of synaptic vesicles, partially preserves baseline firing activity and inhibits amyloid formation (Alhebshi et al., 2013). Several studies have also demonstrated potential efficacy of thymoquinone in the management of PD (Radad et al., 2009; Ebrahimi et al., 2017).

Ginseng, a root of *Panax* species, has long tradition as a medicinal herb in Asian countries. It enhances immune response, improves cognitive functioning, and reduces the risk of dementia. The major active compounds of ginseng are ginsenosides, of which Rb1, Rd, Re and Rg1 are the most studied (Mohd Sairazi and Sirajudeen, 2000). In human neuroblastoma SH-SY5Y cells treated with MPP^+ that induces motor abnormalities similar to PD in animal models, ginsenoside Rg1, an active ingredient of *Panax ginseng,* exhibits neuroprotective effects. Rg1 depletes ROS generation and attenuates JNK and caspase-3 activity, indicating its antioxidative and antiapoptotic properties (Chen et al., 2003). Rg1 also protects hippocampal cells against D-galactose-induced aging in a rat model. It preserves cognitive capacity and hippocampal neurogenesis, increases activity of GSH-Px and SOD, attenuates release of pro-inflammatory cytokines, and suppresses expression of p53 mRNA in the hippocampus of aged rats, altogether modifying p19/p53/p21 signaling pathway (Zhu et al., 2014). Similar results have been obtained in mice, where Rg1 attenuates cognitive decline and senescence of neural stem cells by reducing OS, p53 expression, and Akt/mTOR signaling (Chen et al., 2018a). In SK-N-SH neuroblastoma cells, exposure to H_2O_2 upregulates expression of peptidyl arginine deiminase type 4 (PADI4), a marker of OS response, and decreases expression of estrogen receptor (ER) β. Extract of red ginseng containing all major ginsenosides (Rb1, Rg2, Rg3, Rc, Rb2, Rf, Re, Rd and Rg1) prevents aforementioned changes and inhibits apoptosis by supressing activation of p53, capsase-3, and JNK signaling (Kim et al., 2013).

Bilobalide, a terpenoid from Ginkgo biloba leaves, also attenuates ROS-mediated apoptosis and increases of p53 and Bax expression in PC12 cells (Zhou and Zhu, 2000). In another study, standardized extract of Gingko biloba (EGb761) has counteracted zinc-induced phosphorylation of tau in cultured cortical neurons in a concentration-dependent manner (Kwon et al., 2015). Furthermore, EGb761 has also prevented ROS increase and zinc-induced activation of p38 and GSK-3β (Kwon et al., 2015). In another study, EGb761 has shown protective effect in SK-N-BE neuroblastoma cells against H_2O_2-induced apoptosis. H_2O_2 increases p53 acetylation, Bax/Bcl-2 ratio and PARP-1 cleavage, and these effects have been recently shown to be preventable by Egb761 (Di Meo et al., 2020). Pseudoginsenoside-F11 (PF11), a ginsenoside from *Panax quinquefolium* improves Aβ-induced cognitive impairment in Tg-APPswe/PS1dE9 (APP/PS1) mice. Besides inhibiting expression of Aβ precursor protein (APP), PF11 restores activities of antioxidative enzymes SOD and GSH-Px, and decreases level of lipid peroxidation. In the hippocampus and cortex, PF11 has also demonstrated anti-apoptotic effect by attenuating expression of p53, JNK, and caspase-3 (Wang et al., 2013).

Protosappanin B, a dibenzoxocin derivative from the *Caesalpinia sappan* L., exhibits neuroprotective effects against oxygen-glucose deprivation in PC12 cells. Protosappanin B inhibits cytochrome c release from mytochondria and neuronal apoptosis, and preserves mitochondrial homeostasis by promoting ubiquitin-dependent degradation of p53 protein (Zeng et al. 2015).

Neuroprotective and anti-oxidative effects of myristargenol A, a lignin isolated from *Myristica fragrans*, against glutamate-induced injury of hippocampal HT22 cells is mediated through the suppressed activity of p53 and kinases p38 and JNK, and through an enhanced activity of ERK1/2 (Park et al., 2019). Lycopene, a carotenoid pigment from the red-colored fruits and vegetables, such as tomato, is yet another powerful antioxidant. It inhibits Aβ-induced apoptotic death of SH-SY5Y cells. Among other effects, it reduces expression of p53 and Bax, attenuates ROS production and preserves mitochondrial functioning (Hwang et al., 2017).

Osmotin, a protein isolated from *Nicotiana tabacum*, has been shown to be effective against Aβ-induced memory impairment in mice. Osmotin reduces synaptic deficits, accumulation of Aβ and expression of BACE1, as well as tau hyperphosphorylation by regulating phosphorylation and activity of pAkt and GSK-3β signaling (Ali et al., 2015). Furthermore, osmotin attenuates glutamate-induced excitotoxicity in the cortex and hippocampus of the 7-day-old rats, at least partially via a p53-dependent mechanism. It prevents glutamate receptor activation, attenuates glutamate-mediated production of ROS, DNA fragmentation and synaptic toxicity, and inhibits neuronal apoptosis by activating JNK/PI3K/Akt pathway. At the same time, it reverses glutamate-induced effects on the expression of p53, Bax, Bcl-2, caspase-3, and PARP-1. Lastly, osmotin reverses hippocampal changes in p53 distribution after glutamate exposure (Shah et al., 2014).

Finally, curcumin, a component of the spice turmeric, which is extracted from the rhizome of *Curcuma longa*, is extensively studied as a therapeutic option, particularly as a potential AD-modifying drug. It prevents aggregation of Aβ, restores normal mitochondrial and synaptic function, improves cognitive abilities, and enhances adult neurogenesis (Reddy et al., 2018). Similarly to other health-promoting nutraceuticals, it exhibits multi-target effects: antioxidative, antiapoptotic, and anti-inflammatory (Chen et al., 2018b). Recently, it has been reviewed that curcumin is very effective against oxido-nitrosative stress. It prevents lipid and protein oxidation, and upregulates endogenous anti-oxidative enzymes (Abrahams et al., 2019). Steroidal curcumin derivatives have demonstrated beneficial effects in animal models of AD. In adult female rats, these hybrid agents have increased levels of acetylcholinesterase, glutathione, and Bcl-2, and have decreased levels of p53 and caspase-3 (Elmegeed et al., 2015). As a β-diketone derivative, curcumin effectively chelate metal ions. Metal complexes containing curcumin also possess promising health effects for treatment of AD (Wanninger et al., 2015). Besides inhibiting aggregation of soluble and insoluble Aβ, turmeric extract also reduces levels of phosphorylated tau protein in transgenic Tg2576 mice that over-express Aβ protein (Shytle et al., 2015). *In vitro* study has revealed that curcumin binds to foetal and postnatal human tau isoforms, likely in the microtubule-binding domain (Rane et al., 2017). Through this binding, curcumin prevents formation of β-sheet structure, an initial step in tau assembly, and inhibits tau oligomerization and aggregation. The same study showed that curcumin had disaggregation effect on already formed tau oligomers and filaments (Rane et al., 2017). Curcumin has been also shown to inhibit aggregation of α-synuclein in dopaminergic neurons of lipopolysaccharide-induced PD in rats, and reduce NF-κB activity, formation of NO, promote decline in GSH levels, and decrease iron accumulation in the midbrain of treated animals (Sharma and Nehru, 2018). In dopaminergic SH-SY5Y cells, curcumin prevents 6-OHDA-induced OS and cell death by reducing levels of ROS and p53 phosphorylation, thus restoring Bax/Bcl-2 ratio (Jaisin et al., 2011). Potential contribution of OS is also considered in the pathogenesis of migraine, a common neuropathic pain syndrome. In a study performed on human umbilical vein endothelial cells (HUVECs), pre-treatment with curcumin has improved H_2O_2-induced decrease in the activities of antioxidative enzymes, accompanied with reduction of ROS and MDA level, and attenuation of p53 and other proteins involved in apoptosis, thus indicating that p53-mediated neuroprotective effects of curcumin could be beneficial in a wide range of pathologies (Ouyang et al., 2019).

CONCLUSION

Natural compounds may act as multi-target drugs, particularly in OS conditions. Based on their numerous biological and pharmacological effects, together with a widespread availability and relatively low toxicity, they are considered as promising candidates in the prevention and therapy of neurodegenerative diseases, as well as good precursors for the development of novel therapeutics. It is commonly accepted that a long-term diet enriched in polyphenols (such as Mediterranean-type diet) could have beneficial, health-promoting effects that increase the overall well-being. Besides providing antioxidative effects (direct free radical scavenging, metal chelation, and transcriptional modulations of genes participating in endogenous enzymatic and non-enzymatic antioxidative defence), polyphenolic compounds are important regulators of signaling pathways. Among those pathways, p53 is recognized as being critically involved in determining cell fate in oxidative environment. Hence, polyphenolic modifiers of p53 activity could be promising agents for potential long-term administration or for the development and design of novel neuroprotective drugs. From the numerous studies presented here it is obvious that natural compounds have great potential in targeting p53 pathways. However, further studies are needed to completely elucidate their full potential for human health. For example, depending on the pattern of substituted groups on benzene rings, the extent of the hydroxylation of aglycon and specific modifications of pyran ring, various derivatives of flavonoids could be designed with desired pharmacological activities, together with high bioavailability, that will hopefully bring further improvements in the management of neurodegenerative diseases.

REFERENCES

Abrahams, S., Haylett, W. L., Johnson, G., Carr, J. A., and Bardien, S. (2019). Antioxidant effects of curcumin in models of neurodegeneration, aging, oxidative and nitrosative stress: A review. *Neuroscience*, 406: 1–21. https://doi.org/10.1016/j.neuroscience.2019.02.020.

Ai, Z., Li, C., Li, L., and He, G. (2015). Resveratrol inhibits β-amyloid-induced neuronal apoptosis via regulation of p53 acetylation in PC12 cells. *Molecular medicine reports*, 11(4): 2429–2434. https://doi.org/10.3892/mmr.2014.3034.

Alhebshi, A. H., Gotoh, M., and Suzuki, I. (2013). Thymoquinone protects cultured rat primary neurons against amyloid β-induced neurotoxicity. *Biochemical and biophysical research communications*, 433(4): 362–367. https://doi.org/10.1016/j.bbrc.2012.11.139.

Alavi Naini, S. M., and Soussi-Yanicostas, N. (2015). Tau hyperphosphorylation and oxidative stress, a critical vicious circle in neurodegenerative tauopathies?. *Oxidative medicine and cellular longevity*, 2015, 151979. https://doi.org/10.1155/2015/151979.

Ali, T., Yoon, G. H., Shah, S. A., Lee, H. Y., and Kim, M. O. (2015). Osmotin attenuates amyloid beta-induced memory impairment, tau phosphorylation and neurodegeneration in the mouse hippocampus. *Scientific reports*, 5, 11708. https://doi.org/10.1038/srep11708.

Amanzadeh, E., Esmaeili, A., Abadi, R., Kazemipour, N., Pahlevanneshan, Z., and Beheshti, S. (2019). Quercetin conjugated with superparamagnetic iron oxide nanoparticles improves learning and memory better than free quercetin via interacting with proteins involved in LTP. *Scientific reports*, 9(1), 6876. https://doi.org/10.1038/s41598-019-43345-w.

Anbarasan, T., and Bourdon, J. C. (2019). The emerging landscape of p53 isoforms in physiology, cancer and degenerative diseases. *International journal of molecular sciences*, 20(24), 6257. https://doi.org/10.3390/ijms20246257.

Ashaari, Z., Hadjzadeh, M. A., Hassanzadeh, G., Alizamir, T., Yousefi, B., Keshavarzi, Z., and Mokhtari, T. (2018). The flavone luteolin improves central nervous system disorders by different mechanisms: a review. *Journal of molecular neuroscience: MN*, 65(4): 491–506. https://doi.org/10.1007/s12031-018-1094-2.

Ayaz, M., Sadiq, A., Junaid, M., Ullah, F., Ovais, M., Ullah, I., Ahmed, J., and Shahid, M. (2019). Flavonoids as prospective neuroprotectants and their therapeutic propensity in aging associated neurological disorders. *Frontiers in aging neuroscience*, 11, 155. https://doi.org/10.3389/fnagi.2019.00155.

Bao, D., Wang, J., Pang, X., and Liu, H. (2017). Protective effect of quercetin against qxidative stress-induced cytotoxicity in rat pheochromocytoma (PC-12) cells. *Molecules (Basel, Switzerland)*, 22(7), 1122. https://doi.org/10.3390/molecules22071122.

Barone, E., Cenini, G., Sultana, R., Di Domenico, F., Fiorini, A., Perluigi, M., Noel, T., Wang, C., Mancuso, C., St Clair, D. K., and Butterfield, D. A. (2012). Lack of p53 decreases basal oxidative stress levels in the brain through upregulation of thioredoxin-1, biliverdin reductase-A, manganese superoxide dismutase, and nuclear factor kappa-B. *Antioxidants & redox signaling*, 16(12): 1407–1420. https://doi.org/10.1089/ars.2011.4124.

Bastianetto, S., Ménard, C., and Quirion, R. (2015). Neuroprotective action of resveratrol. *Biochimica et biophysica acta*, 1852(6): 1195–1201. https://doi.org/10.1016/j.bbadis.2014.09.011.

Bonda, D. J., Wang, X., Perry, G., Nunomura, A., Tabaton, M., Zhu, X., and Smith, M. A. (2010). Oxidative stress in Alzheimer disease: a possibility for prevention. *Neuropharmacology*, 59(4-5): 290–294. https://doi.org/10.1016/j.neuropharm.2010.04.005.

Bourdon J. C. (2007). p53 and its isoforms in cancer. *British journal of cancer*, 97(3): 277–282. https://doi.org/10.1038/sj.bjc.6603886.

Bykov, V. J., Lambert, J. M., Hainaut, P., and Wiman, K. G. (2009). Mutant p53 rescue and modulation of p53 redox state. *Cell cycle (Georgetown, Tex.)*, 8(16): 2509–2517. https://doi.org/10.4161/cc.8.16.9382.

Çelik, H., Kandemir, F. M., Caglayan, C., Özdemir, S., Çomaklı, S., Kucukler, S., and Yardım, A. (2020). Neuroprotective effect of rutin against colistin-induced oxidative stress, inflammation and apoptosis in rat brain associated with the CREB/BDNF expressions. *Molecular biology reports*, 47(3): 2023–2034. https://doi.org/10.1007/s11033-020-05302-z.

Chang, J. R., Ghafouri, M., Mukerjee, R., Bagashev, A., Chabrashvili, T., and Sawaya, B. E. (2012). Role of p53 in neurodegenerative diseases. *Neurodegenerative diseases*, 9(2): 68–80. https://doi.org/10.1159/000329999.

Chatoo, W., Abdouh, M., and Bernier, G. (2011). p53 pro-oxidant activity in the central nervous system: implication in aging and neurodegenerative diseases. *Antioxidants & redox signaling*, 15(6): 1729–1737. https://doi.org/10.1089/ars.2010.3610.

Cheignon, C., Tomas, M., Bonnefont-Rousselot, D., Faller, P., Hureau, C., and Collin, F. (2018). Oxidative stress and the amyloid beta peptide in Alzheimer's disease. *Redox biology*, 14: 450–464. https://doi.org/10.1016/j.redox.2017.10.014.

Chen, J. X., and Yan, S. D. (2007). Amyloid-beta-induced mitochondrial dysfunction. *Journal of Alzheimer's disease: JAD*, 12(2): 177–184. https://doi.org/10.3233/jad-2007-12208.

Chen, L., Yao, H., Chen, X., Wang, Z., Xiang, Y., Xia, J., Liu, Y., and Wang, Y. (2018a). Ginsenoside Rg1 decreases oxidative stress and down-regulates Akt/mTOR signalling to attenuate cognitive impairment in mice and senescence of neural stem cells induced by D-galactose. *Neurochemical research*, 43(2): 430–440. https://doi.org/10.1007/s11064-017-2438-y.

Chen, M., Du, Z. Y., Zheng, X., Li, D. L., Zhou, R. P., and Zhang, K. (2018b). Use of curcumin in diagnosis, prevention, and treatment of Alzheimer's disease. *Neural regeneration research*, 13(4): 742–752. https://doi.org/10.4103/1673-5374.230303.

Chen, X. C., Fang, F., Zhu, Y. G., Chen, L. M., Zhou, Y. C., and Chen, Y. (2003). Protective effect of ginsenoside Rg1 on MPP^+-induced apoptosis in SHSY5Y cells. *Journal of neural transmission (Vienna, Austria: 1996)*, 110(8), 835–845. https://doi.org/10.1007/s00702-003-0005-y.

Cheng, H. Y., Hsieh, M. T., Tsai, F. S., Wu, C. R., Chiu, C. S., Lee, M. M., Xu, H. X., Zhao, Z. Z., and Peng, W. H. (2010). Neuroprotective effect of luteolin on amyloid beta protein (25-35)-induced toxicity in cultured rat cortical neurons. *Phytotherapy research: PTR*, 24 Suppl 1: S102–S108. https://doi.org/10.1002/ptr.2940.

Corpas, R., Griñán-Ferré, C., Rodríguez-Farré, E., Pallàs, M., and Sanfeliu, C. (2019). Resveratrol induces brain resilience against Alzheimer neurodegeneration through proteostasis enhancement. *Molecular neurobiology*, 56(2): 1502–1516. https://doi.org/10.1007/s12035-018-1157-y.

Costa, L. G., Garrick, J. M., Roquè, P. J., and Pellacani, C. (2016). Mechanisms of neuroprotection by quercetin: counteracting oxidative stress and more. *Oxidative medicine and cellular longevity*, 2016, 2986796. https://doi.org/10.1155/2016/2986796.

Culmsee, C., Zhu, X., Yu, Q. S., Chan, S. L., Camandola, S., Guo, Z., Greig, N. H., and Mattson, M. P. (2001). A synthetic inhibitor of p53 protects neurons against death induced by ischemic and excitotoxic insults, and amyloid beta-peptide. *Journal of neurochemistry*, 77(1): 220–228. https://doi.org/10.1046/j.1471-4159.2001.t01-1-00220.x.

Dai, C. Q., Luo, T. T., Luo, S. C., Wang, J. Q., Wang, S. M., Bai, Y. H., Yang, Y. L., and Wang, Y. Y. (2016). p53 and mitochondrial dysfunction: novel insight of neurodegenerative diseases. *Journal of bioenergetics and biomembranes*, 48(4): 337–347. https://doi.org/10.1007/s10863-016-9669-5.

Darendelioglu E. (2020). Neuroprotective effects of chrysin on diclofenac-induced apoptosis in SH-SY5Y cells. *Neurochemical research*, 45(5): 1064–1071. https://doi.org/10.1007/s11064-020-02982-8.

Davinelli, S., Maes, M., Corbi, G., Zarrelli, A., Willcox, D. C., and Scapagnini, G. (2016). Dietary phytochemicals and neuro-inflammaging: from mechanistic insights to translational challenges. *Immunity & ageing: I & A*, 13, 16. https://doi.org/10.1186/s12979-016-0070-3.

Diana, A., Šimić, G., Sinforiani, E., Orrù, N., Pichiri, G., and Bono, G. (2008) Mitochondria morphology and DNA content upon sublethal exposure to β-amyloid$_{1\text{-}42}$ peptide. *Collegium Antropologicum*, 32 (Suppl. 1): 51-58. PMID 18405058.

Di Domenico, F., Cenini, G., Sultana, R., Perluigi, M., Uberti, D., Memo, M., and Butterfield, D. A. (2009). Glutathionylation of the pro-apoptotic protein p53 in Alzheimer's disease brain: implications for AD pathogenesis. *Neurochemical research*, 34(4): 727–733. https://doi.org/10.1007/s11064-009-9924-9.

Di Giovanni, S., Knights, C. D., Rao, M., Yakovlev, A., Beers, J., Catania, J., Avantaggiati, M. L., and Faden, A. I. (2006). The tumor suppressor protein p53 is required for neurite outgrowth and axon regeneration. *The EMBO journal*, 25(17): 4084–4096. https://doi.org/10.1038/sj.emboj.7601292.

Di Giovanni, S., and Rathore, K. (2012). p53-Dependent pathways in neurite outgrowth and axonal regeneration. *Cell and tissue research*, 349(1): 87–95. https://doi.org/10.1007/s00441-011-1292-5.

Di Meo, F., Cuciniello, R., Margarucci, S., Bergamo, P., Petillo, O., Peluso, G., Filosa, S., and Crispi, S. (2020). *Ginkgo biloba* prevents oxidative stress-induced apoptosis blocking p53 activation in neuroblastoma cells. *Antioxidants (Basel, Switzerland)*, 9(4): 279. https://doi.org/10.3390/antiox9040279.

Ebrahimi, S. S., Oryan, S., Izadpanah, E., and Hassanzadeh K. (2017) Thymoquinone exerts neuroprotective effect in animal model of Parkinson's disease. *Toxicology letters*, 276: 108-114. https://doi.org/10.1016/j.toxlet.2017.05.018.

Eizenberg, O., Faber-Elman, A., Gottlieb, E., Oren, M., Rotter, V., and Schwartz, M. (1996). p53 plays a regulatory role in differentiation and apoptosis of central nervous system-associated cells. *Molecular and cellular biology*, 16(9): 5178–5185. https://doi.org/10.1128/mcb.16.9.5178.

El-Horany, H. E., El-Latif, R. N., ElBatsh, M. M., and Emam, M. N. (2016). Ameliorative effect of quercetin on neurochemical and behavioral deficits in rotenone rat model of Parkinson's disease: modulating autophagy (Quercetin on experimental Parkinson's disease). *Journal of biochemical and molecular toxicology*, 30(7): 360–369. https://doi.org/10.1002/jbt.21821.

Elmegeed, G. A., Ahmed, H. H., Hashash, M. A., Abd-Elhalim, M. M., and El-kady, D. S. (2015). Synthesis of novel steroidal curcumin derivatives as anti-Alzheimer's disease candidates: Evidences-based on *in vivo* study. *Steroids*, 101: 78–89. https://doi.org/10.1016/j.steroids.2015.06.003.

Engel, T., Murphy, B. M., Hatazaki, S., Jimenez-Mateos, E. M., Concannon, C. G., Woods, I., Prehn, J. H., and Henshall, D. C. (2010). Reduced hippocampal damage and epileptic seizures after status epilepticus in mice lacking proapoptotic Puma. *FASEB journal: official publication of the Federation of American Societies for Experimental Biology*, 24(3): 853–861. https://doi.org/10.1096/fj.09-145870.

Fan, Q. D., Wu, G., and Liu, Z. R. (2014). Dynamics of posttranslational modifications of p53. *Computational and mathematical methods in medicine*, 2014, 245610. https://doi.org/10.1155/2014/245610.

Farmer, K. M., Ghag, G., Puangmalai, N., Montalbano, M., Bhatt, N., and Kayed, R. (2020). P53 aggregation, interactions with tau, and impaired DNA damage response in Alzheimer's disease. *Acta neuropathologica communications*, 8(1): 132. https://doi.org/10.1186/s40478-020-01012-6.

Feng, X., Liang, N., Zhu, D., Gao, Q., Peng, L., Dong, H., Yue, Q., Liu, H., Bao, L., Zhang, J., Hao, J., Gao, Y., Yu, X., and Sun, J. (2013). Resveratrol inhibits β-amyloid-induced neuronal apoptosis through regulation of SIRT1-ROCK1 signaling pathway. *PloS one*, 8(3), e59888. https://doi.org/10.1371/journal.pone.0059888.

Feng, Y., Liu, T., Dong, S. Y., Guo, Y. J., Jankovic, J., Xu, H., and Wu, Y. C. (2015). Rotenone affects p53 transcriptional activity and apoptosis via targeting SIRT1 and H3K9 acetylation in SH-SY5Y cells. *Journal of neurochemistry*, 134(4): 668–676. https://doi.org/10.1111/jnc.13172.

Fischer, N. W., Prodeus, A., Malkin, D., & Gariépy, J. (2016). p53 oligomerization status modulates cell fate decisions between growth, arrest and apoptosis. *Cell cycle (Georgetown, Tex.)*, 15(23): 3210–3219. https://doi.org/10.1080/15384101.2016.1241917.

Fu, J., Sun, H., Zhang, Y., Xu, W., Wang, C., Fang, Y., and Zhao, J. (2018). Neuroprotective effects of luteolin against spinal cord ischemia-reperfusion injury by attenuation of oxidative stress, inflammation, and apoptosis. *Journal of medicinal food*, 21(1): 13–20. https://doi.org/10.1089/jmf.2017.4021.

Goiran, T., Duplan, E., Rouland, L., El Manaa, W., Lauritzen, I., Dunys, J., You, H., Checler, F., and Alves da Costa, C. (2018). Nuclear p53-mediated repression of autophagy involves PINK1 transcriptional down-regulation. *Cell death and differentiation*, 25(5): 873–884. https://doi.org/10.1038/s41418-017-0016-0.

Gomes, B., Silva, J., Romeiro, C., Dos Santos, S. M., Rodrigues, C. A., Gonçalves, P. R., Sakai, J. T., Mendes, P., Varela, E., and Monteiro, M. C. (2018). Neuroprotective mechanisms of resveratrol in Alzheimer's disease: ryole of SIRT1. *Oxidative medicine and cellular longevity*, 2018: 8152373. https://doi.org/10.1155/2018/8152373.

Gong, Y. S., Guo, J., Hu, K., Gao, Y. Q., Xie, B. J., Sun, Z. D., Yang, E. N., and Hou, F. L. (2016). Ameliorative effect of lotus seedpod proanthocyanidins on cognitive impairment and brain aging induced by D-galactose. *Experimental gerontology*, 74: 21–28. https://doi.org/10.1016/j.exger.2015.11.020.

Guo, C., Sun, L., Chen, X. and Zhang, D. (2013a). Oxidative stress, mitochondrial damage and neurodegenerative diseases. *Neural regeneration research*, 8(21): 2003–2014. https://doi.org/10.3969/j.issn.1673-5374.2013.21.009.

Guo, D. J., Li, F., Yu, P. H., and Chan, S. W. (2013b). Neuroprotective effects of luteolin against apoptosis induced by 6-hydroxydopamine on rat pheochromocytoma PC12 cells. *Pharmaceutical biology*, 51(2): 190–196. https://doi.org/10.3109/13880209.2012.716852.

Guo, H., Kong, S., Chen, W., Dai, Z., Lin, T., Su, J., Li, S., Xie, Q., Su, Z., Xu, Y., and Lai, X. (2014). Apigenin mediated protection of OGD-evoked neuron-like injury in differentiated PC12 cells. *Neurochemical research*, 39(11): 2197–2210. https://doi.org/10.1007/s11064-014-1421-0.

Guo, T., Noble, W., and Hanger, D. P. (2017). Roles of tau protein in health and disease. *Acta neuropathologica*, 133(5): 665–704. https://doi.org/10.1007/s00401-017-1707-9.

Hafner, A., Bulyk, M. L., Jambhekar, A., and Lahav, G. (2019). The multiple mechanisms that regulate p53 activity and cell fate. *Nature reviews.*

Molecular cell biology, 20(4): 199–210. https://doi.org/10.1038/s41580-019-0110-x.

Han, J. Y., Ahn, S. Y., Kim, C. S., Yoo, S. K., Kim, S. K., Kim, H. C., Hong, J. T., and Oh, K. W. (2012). Protection of apigenin against kainate-induced excitotoxicity by anti-oxidative effects. *Biological & pharmaceutical bulletin*, 35(9): 1440–1446. https://doi.org/10.1248/bpb.b110686.

Holley, A. K., Dhar, S. K., and St Clair, D. K. (2010). Manganese superoxide dismutase vs. p53: regulation of mitochondrial ROS. *Mitochondrion*, 10(6): 649–661. https://doi.org/10.1016/j.mito.2010.06.003.

Hooper, C., Meimaridou, E., Tavassoli, M., Melino, G., Lovestone, S., and Killick, R. (2007). p53 is upregulated in Alzheimer's disease and induces tau phosphorylation in HEK293a cells. *Neuroscience letters*, 418(1): 34–37. https://doi.org/10.1016/j.neulet.2007.03.026.

Hoshino, A., Mita, Y., Okawa, Y., Ariyoshi, M., Iwai-Kanai, E., Ueyama, T., Ikeda, K., Ogata, T., and Matoba, S. (2013). Cytosolic p53 inhibits Parkin-mediated mitophagy and promotes mitochondrial dysfunction in the mouse heart. *Nature communications*, 4: 2308. https://doi.org/10.1038/ncomms3308.

Hu, L. W., Yen, J. H., Shen, Y. T., Wu, K. Y., and Wu, M. J. (2014). Luteolin modulates 6-hydroxydopamine-induced transcriptional changes of stress response pathways in PC12 cells. *PloS one*, 9(5): e97880. https://doi.org/10.1371/journal.pone.0097880.

Huang, Y. N., Yang, L. Y., Greig, N. H., Wang, Y. C., Lai, C. C., and Wang, J. Y. (2018). Neuroprotective effects of pifithrin-α against traumatic brain injury in the striatum through suppression of neuroinflammation, oxidative stress, autophagy, and apoptosis. *Scientific reports*, 8(1): 2368. https://doi.org/10.1038/s41598-018-19654-x.

Hwang, S., Lim, J. W., and Kim, H. (2017). Inhibitory effect of lycopene on amyloid-β-induced apoptosis in neuronal cells. *Nutrients*, 9(8): 883. https://doi.org/10.3390/nu9080883.

Ismail, N., Ismail, M., Azmi, N. H., Abu Bakar, M. F., Basri, H., and Abdullah, M. A. (2016). Modulation of hydrogen peroxide-induced oxidative stress in human neuronal cells by thymoquinone-rich fraction and thymoquinone via transcriptomic regulation of antioxidant and apoptotic signaling genes. *Oxidative medicine and cellular longevity*, 2016: 2528935. https://doi.org/10.1155/2016/2528935.

Jaisin, Y., Thampithak, A., Meesarapee, B., Ratanachamnong, P., Suksamrarn, A., Phivthong-Ngam, L., Phumala-Morales, N., Chongthammakun, S., Govitrapong, P., and Sanvarinda, Y. (2011). Curcumin I protects the dopaminergic cell line SH-SY5Y from 6-hydroxydopamine-induced neurotoxicity through attenuation of p53-mediated apoptosis. *Neuroscience letters*, 489(3): 192–196. https://doi.org/10.1016/j.neulet.2010.12.014.

Javed, H., Khan, M. M., Ahmad, A., Vaibhav, K., Ahmad, M. E., Khan, A., Ashafaq, M., Islam, F., Siddiqui, M. S., Safhi, M. M., and Islam, F. (2012). Rutin prevents cognitive impairments by ameliorating oxidative stress and neuroinflammation in rat model of sporadic dementia of Alzheimer type. *Neuroscience*, 210: 340–352. https://doi.org/10.1016/j.neuroscience.2012.02.046.

Jazvinšćak Jembrek, M., Čipak Gašparović, A., Vuković, L., Vlainić, J., Žarković, N., and Oršolić, N. (2012a). Quercetin supplementation: insight into the potentially harmful outcomes of neurodegenerative prevention. *Naunyn-Schmiedeberg's archives of pharmacology*, 385(12): 1185–1197. https://doi.org/10.1007/s00210-012-0799-y.

Jazvinšćak Jembrek, M., Babić, M., Pivac, N., Hof., P. R., and Šimić, G. (2013) Hyperphosphorylation of tau by GSK-3β in Alzheimer's disease: the interaction of Aβ and sphingolipid mediators as a therapeutic target. *Translational Neuroscience*, 4(4): 466-476. https://doi.org/10.2478/s13380-013-0144-z.

Jazvinšćak Jembrek, M., Hof, P. R., and Šimić, G. (2015). Ceramides in Alzheimer's disease: key mediators of neuronal apoptosis induced by oxidative stress and Aβ accumulation. *Oxidative medicine and cellular longevity*, 2015: 346783. https://doi.org/10.1155/2015/346783.

Jazvinšćak Jembrek, M., Slade, N., Hof, P. R., and Šimić, G. (2018a). The interactions of p53 with tau and Aß as potential therapeutic targets for Alzheimer's disease. *Progress in neurobiology*, 168: 104–127. https://doi.org/10.1016/j.pneurobio.2018.05.001.

Jazvinšćak Jembrek, M., Vlainić, J., Čadež, V., and Šegota, S. (2018b). Atomic force microscopy reveals new biophysical markers for monitoring subcellular changes in oxidative injury: Neuroprotective effects of quercetin at the nanoscale. *PloS one*, *13*(10): e0200119. https://doi.org/10.1371/journal.pone.0200119.

Jazvinšćak Jembrek, M., Vlainić, J., Radovanović, V., Erhardt, J., and Oršolić, N. (2014). Effects of copper overload in P19 neurons: impairment of glutathione redox homeostasis and crosstalk between caspase and calpain protease systems in ROS-induced apoptosis. *Biometals: an international journal on the role of metal ions in biology, biochemistry, and medicine*, 27(6): 1303–1322. https://doi.org/10.1007/s10534-014-9792-x.

Jazvinšćak Jembrek, M., Vuković, L., Puhović, J., Erhardt, J., and Oršolić, N. (2012b). Neuroprotective effect of quercetin against hydrogen peroxide-induced oxidative injury in P19 neurons. *Journal of molecular neuroscience*, 47(2): 286–299. https://doi.org/10.1007/s12031-012-9737-1

Jordán, J., Galindo, M. F., Prehn, J. H., Weichselbaum, R. R., Beckett, M., Ghadge, G. D., Roos, R. P., Leiden, J. M., and Miller, R. J. (1997). p53 expression induces apoptosis in hippocampal pyramidal neuron cultures. *The Journal of neuroscience: the official journal of the Society for Neuroscience*, 17(4): 1397–1405. https://doi.org/10.1523/JNEUROSCI.17-04-01397.1997.

Jung, J. Y., Han, C. R., Jeong, Y. J., Kim, H. J., Lim, H. S., Lee, K. H., Park, H. O., Oh, W. M., Kim, S. H., and Kim, W. J. (2007). Epigallocatechin gallate inhibits nitric oxide-induced apoptosis in rat PC12 cells. *Neuroscience letters*, 411(3): 222–227. https://doi.org/10.1016/j.neulet.2006.09.089.

Kang, K. A., Piao, M. J., Hyun, Y. J., Zhen, A. X., Cho, S. J., Ahn, M. J., Yi, J. M., and Hyun, J. W. (2019). Luteolin promotes apoptotic cell death via upregulation of Nrf2 expression by DNA demethylase and the interaction of Nrf2 with p53 in human colon cancer cells. *Experimental & molecular medicine*, 51(4): 1–14. https://doi.org/10.1038/s12276-019-0238-y.

Katsel, P., Tan, W., Fam, P., Purohit, D. P., and Haroutunian, V. (2013). Cell cycle checkpoint abnormalities during dementia: A plausible association with the loss of protection against oxidative stress in Alzheimer's disease. *PloS one*, 8(7): e68361. https://doi.org/10.1371/journal.pone.0068361.

Khan, A., Vaibhav, K., Javed, H., Khan, M. M., Tabassum, R., Ahmed, M. E., Srivastava, P., Khuwaja, G., Islam, F., Siddiqui, M. S., Safhi, M. M., and Islam, F. (2012). Attenuation of Aβ-induced neurotoxicity by thymoquinone via inhibition of mitochondrial dysfunction and oxidative stress. *Molecular and cellular biochemistry*, 369(1-2): 55–65. https://doi.org/10.1007/s11010-012-1368-x.

Khan, H., Ullah, H., Aschner, M., Cheang, W. S., and Akkol, E. K. (2019a). Neuroprotective effects of quercetin in Alzheimer's disease. *Biomolecules*, 10(1): 59. https://doi.org/10.3390/biom10010059.

Khan, M. M., Ahmad, A., Ishrat, T., Khuwaja, G., Srivastawa, P., Khan, M. B., Raza, S. S., Javed, H., Vaibhav, K., Khan, A., and Islam, F. (2009). Rutin protects the neural damage induced by transient focal ischemia in rats. *Brain research*, 1292: 123–135. https://doi.org/10.1016/j.brainres.2009.07.026.

Khan, M. S., Ali, T., Kim, M. W., Jo, M. H., Chung, J. I., and Kim, M. O. (2019b). Anthocyanins improve hippocampus-dependent memory function and prevent neurodegeneration via JNK/Akt/GSK3β signaling in LPS-treated adult mice. *Molecular neurobiology*, 56(1): 671–687. https://doi.org/10.1007/s12035-018-1101-1.

Khoury, M. P., and Bourdon, J. C. (2011). p53 Isoforms: an intracellular microprocessor?. *Genes & cancer*, 2(4): 453–465. https://doi.org/10.1177/1947601911408893.

Kim, D., Nguyen, M. D., Dobbin, M. M., Fischer, A., Sananbenesi, F., Rodgers, J. T., Delalle, I., Baur, J. A., Sui, G., Armour, S. M., Puigserver, P., Sinclair, D. A., and Tsai, L. H. (2007). SIRT1 deacetylase protects against neurodegeneration in models for Alzheimer's disease and amyotrophic lateral sclerosis. *The EMBO journal*, 26(13): 3169–3179. https://doi.org/10.1038/sj.emboj.7601758.

Kim, E. H., Kim, I. H., Lee, M. J., Thach Nguyen, C., Ha, J. A., Lee, S. C., Choi, S., Choi, K. T., Pyo, S., and Rhee, D. K. (2013). Anti-oxidative stress effect of red ginseng in the brain is mediated by peptidyl arginine deiminase type IV (PADI4) repression via estrogen receptor (ER) β up-regulation. *Journal of ethnopharmacology*, 148(2): 474–485. https://doi.org/10.1016/j.jep.2013.04.041.

Kim, G. H., Kim, J. E., Rhie, S. J., and Yoon, S. (2015). The role of oxidative stress in neurodegenerative diseases. *Experimental neurobiology*, 24(4): 325–340. https://doi.org/10.5607/en.2015.24.4.325.

Kitamura, Y., Shimohama, S., Kamoshima, W., Matsuoka, Y., Nomura, Y., and Taniguchi, T. (1997). Changes of p53 in the brains of patients with Alzheimer's disease. *Biochemical and biophysical research communications*, 232(2): 418–421. https://doi.org/10.1006/bbrc.1997.6301.

Kong, Y., Li, K., Fu, T., Wan, C., Zhang, D., Song, H., Zhang, Y., Liu, N., Gan, Z., and Yuan, L. (2016). Quercetin ameliorates Aβ toxicity in Drosophila AD model by modulating cell cycle-related protein expression. *Oncotarget*, 7(42): 67716–67731. https://doi.org/10.18632/oncotarget.11963.

Kulasekaran, G., and Ganapasam, S. (2015). Neuroprotective efficacy of naringin on 3-nitropropionic acid-induced mitochondrial dysfunction through the modulation of Nrf2 signaling pathway in PC12 cells. *Molecular and cellular biochemistry*, 409(1-2): 199–211. https://doi.org/10.1007/s11010-015-2525-9.

Kumar, S., Krishnakumar, V. G., Morya, V., Gupta, S., and Datta, B. (2019). Nanobiocatalyst facilitated aglycosidic quercetin as a potent inhibitor of tau protein aggregation. *International journal of biological macromolecules*, 138: 168–180. https://doi.org/10.1016/j.ijbiomac.2019.07.081.

Kwon, K. J., Lee, E. J., Cho, K. S., Cho, D. H., Shin, C. Y., and Han, S. H. (2015). Ginkgo biloba extract (Egb761) attenuates zinc-induced tau phosphorylation at Ser262 by regulating GSK3β activity in rat primary cortical neurons. *Food & function*, 6(6): 2058–2067. https://doi.org/10.1039/c5fo00219b.

Lacroix, M., Riscal, R., Arena, G., Linares, L. K., and Le Cam, L. (2020). Metabolic functions of the tumor suppressor p53: Implications in normal physiology, metabolic disorders, and cancer. *Molecular metabolism*, 33: 2–22. https://doi.org/10.1016/j.molmet.2019.10.002.

Lanni, C., Nardinocchi, L., Puca, R., Stanga, S., Uberti, D., Memo, M., Govoni, S., D'Orazi, G., and Racchi, M. (2010). Homeodomain interacting protein kinase 2: a target for Alzheimer's beta amyloid leading to misfolded p53 and inappropriate cell survival. *PloS One*, 5(4): e10171. https://doi.org/10.1371/journal.pone.0010171.

Lee, J. T., and Gu, W. (2013). SIRT1: regulator of p53 deacetylation. *Genes & cancer*, 4(3-4): 112–117. https://doi.org/10.1177/1947601913484496.

Levites, Y., Amit, T., Youdim, M. B., and Mandel, S. (2002). Involvement of protein kinase C activation and cell survival/ cell cycle genes in green tea polyphenol (-)-epigallocatechin 3-gallate neuroprotective action. *The Journal of biological chemistry*, 277(34): 30574–30580. https://doi.org/10.1074/jbc.M202832200.

Li, B. Y., Yuan, Y. H., Hu, J. F., Zhao, Q., Zhang, D. M., and Chen, N. H. (2011). Protective effect of Bu-7, a flavonoid extracted from Clausena lansium, against rotenone injury in PC12 cells. *Acta pharmacologica Sinica*, 32(11): 1321–1326. https://doi.org/10.1038/aps.2011.119.

Liang, Y., Liu, J., and Feng, Z. (2013). The regulation of cellular metabolism by tumor suppressor p53. *Cell & bioscience*, 3(1): 9. https://doi.org/10.1186/2045-3701-3-9.

Liu, B., Chen, Y., and St Clair, D. K. (2008). ROS and p53: a versatile partnership. *Free radical biology & medicine*, 44(8): 1529–1535. https://doi.org/10.1016/j.freeradbiomed.2008.01.011.

Liu, D., and Xu, Y. (2011). p53, oxidative stress, and aging. *Antioxidants & redox signaling*, 15(6): 1669–1678. https://doi.org/10.1089/ars.2010.3644.

Liu, J., Zhang, C., Hu, W., and Feng, Z. (2015). Tumor suppressor p53 and its mutants in cancer metabolism. *Cancer letters*, 356(2 Pt A): 197–203. https://doi.org/10.1016/j.canlet.2013.12.025.

Liu, Z., Zhou, T., Ziegler, A. C., Dimitrion, P., and Zuo, L. (2017). Oxidative stress in neurodegenerative diseases: from molecular mechanisms to clinical applications. *Oxidative medicine and cellular longevity*, 2017: 2525967. https://doi.org/10.1155/2017/2525967.

Ma, H., Johnson, S. L., Liu, W., DaSilva, N. A., Meschwitz, S., Dain, J. A., and Seeram, N. P. (2018a). Evaluation of polyphenol anthocyanin-enriched extracts of blackberry, black raspberry, blueberry, cranberry, red raspberry, and strawberry for free radical scavenging, reactive carbonyl species trapping, anti-glycation, anti-β-amyloid aggregation, and microglial neuroprotective effects. *International journal of molecular sciences*, 19(2): 461. https://doi.org/10.3390/ijms19020461.

Ma, J., Gao, S. S., Yang, H. J., Wang, M., Cheng, B. F., Feng, Z. W., and Wang, L. (2018b). Neuroprotective effects of proanthocyanidins, natural flavonoids derived from plants, on rotenone-induced oxidative stress and apoptotic cell death in human neuroblastoma SH-SY5Y cells. *Frontiers in neuroscience*, 12: 369. https://doi.org/10.3389/fnins.2018.00369.

Maan, G., Sikdar, B., Kumar, A., Shukla, R., and Mishra, A. (2020). Role of flavonoids in neurodegenerative diseases: limitations and future perspectives. *Current topics in medicinal chemistry*, 20(13): 1169–1194. https://doi.org/10.2174/1568026620666200416085330.

Maher P. (2019). The potential of flavonoids for the treatment of neurodegenerative diseases. *International journal of molecular sciences*, 20(12): 3056. https://doi.org/10.3390/ijms20123056.

Mancini, F., Pieroni, L., Monteleone, V., Lucà, R., Fici, L., Luca, E., Urbani, A., Xiong, S., Soddu, S., Masetti, R., Lozano, G., Pontecorvi, A., and Moretti, F. (2016). MDM4/HIPK2/p53 cytoplasmic assembly uncovers coordinated repression of molecules with anti-apoptotic activity during early DNA damage response. *Oncogene*, 35(2): 228–240. https://doi.org/10.1038/onc.2015.76.

Marcel, V., Petit, I., Murray-Zmijewski, F., Goullet de Rugy, T., Fernandes, K., Meuray, V., Diot, A., Lane, D. P., Aberdam, D., and Bourdon, J. C. (2012). Diverse p63 and p73 isoforms regulate Δ133p53 expression through modulation of the internal TP53 promoter activity. *Cell death and differentiation*, 19(5): 816–826. https://doi.org/10.1038/cdd. 2011.152.

Merlo, P., Frost, B., Peng, S., Yang, Y. J., Park, P. J., and Feany, M. (2014). p53 prevents neurodegeneration by regulating synaptic genes. *Proceedings of the National Academy of Sciences of the United States of America*, 111(50): 18055–18060. https://doi.org/10.1073/pnas. 1419083111.

Mohd Sairazi, N. S., and Sirajudeen, K. (2020). Natural products and their bioactive compounds: neuroprotective potentials against neurodegenerative diseases. *Evidence-based complementary and alternative medicine: eCAM*, 2020: 6565396. https://doi.org/10.1155/ 2020/6565396.

Moll, U. M., and Slade, N. (2004). p63 and p73: roles in development and tumor formation. *Molecular cancer research: MCR*, 2(7): 371–386.

Morrison, R. S., and Kinoshita, Y. (2000). The role of p53 in neuronal cell death. *Cell death and differentiation*, 7(10): 868–879. https://doi.org/10.1038/sj.cdd.4400741.

Morrison, R. S., Wenzel, H. J., Kinoshita, Y., Robbins, C. A., Donehower, L. A., and Schwartzkroin, P. A. (1996). Loss of the p53 tumor suppressor gene protects neurons from kainate-induced cell death. *The Journal of neuroscience: the official journal of the Society for Neuroscience*, 16(4): 1337–1345. https://doi.org/10.1523/ JNEUROSCI.16-04-01337.1996.

Mossmann, D., Vögtle, F. N., Taskin, A. A., Teixeira, P. F., Ring, J., Burkhart, J. M., Burger, N., Pinho, C. M., Tadic, J., Loreth, D., Graff, C., Metzger, F., Sickmann, A., Kretz, O., Wiedemann, N., Zahedi, R. P., Madeo, F., Glaser, E., and Meisinger, C. (2014). Amyloid-β peptide induces mitochondrial dysfunction by inhibition of preprotein maturation. *Cell metabolism*, 20(4): 662–669. https://doi.org/10.1016/ j.cmet.2014.07.024.

Multhaup, G., Scheuermann, S., Schlicksupp, A., Simons, A., Strauss, M., Kemmling, A., Oehler, C., Cappai, R., Pipkorn, R., and Bayer, T. A. (2002). Possible mechanisms of APP-mediated oxidative stress in

Alzheimer's disease. *Free radical biology & medicine*, 33(1): 45–51. https://doi.org/10.1016/s0891-5849(02)00806-7.

Murray-Zmijewski, F., Lane, D. P., and Bourdon, J. C. (2006). p53/p63/p73 isoforms: an orchestra of isoforms to harmonise cell differentiation and response to stress. *Cell death and differentiation*, 13(6): 962–972. https://doi.org/10.1038/sj.cdd.4401914.

Nakanishi, A., Minami, A., Kitagishi, Y., Ogura, Y., and Matsuda, S. (2015). BRCA1 and p53 tumor suppressor molecules in Alzheimer's disease. *International journal of molecular sciences*, 16(2): 2879–2892. https://doi.org/10.3390/ijms16022879.

Neema, M., Navarro-Quiroga, I., Chechlacz, M., Gilliams-Francis, K., Liu, J., Lamonica, K., Lin, S. L., and Naegele, J. R. (2005). DNA damage and nonhomologous end joining in excitotoxicity: neuroprotective role of DNA-PKcs in kainic acid-induced seizures. *Hippocampus*, 15(8): 1057–1071. https://doi.org/10.1002/hipo.20123.

Oliveira, A. M., Cardoso, S. M., Ribeiro, M., Seixas, R. S., Silva, A. M., and Rego, A. C. (2015). Protective effects of 3-alkyl luteolin derivatives are mediated by Nrf2 transcriptional activity and decreased oxidative stress in Huntington's disease mouse striatal cells. *Neurochemistry international*, 91: 1–12. https://doi.org/10.1016/j.neuint.2015.10.004.

Okawara, M., Katsuki, H., Kurimoto, E., Shibata, H., Kume, T., and Akaike, A. (2007). Resveratrol protects dopaminergic neurons in midbrain slice culture from multiple insults. *Biochemical pharmacology*, 73: 550-560. https://doi.org/10.1016/j.bcp.2006.11.003.

Ouyang, J., Li, R., Shi, H., and Zhong, J. (2019). Curcumin protects human umbilical vein endothelial cells against H_2O_2-induced cell injury. *Pain research & management*, 2019, 3173149. https://doi.org/10.1155/2019/3173149.

Park, J. H., Ko, J., Hwang, J., and Koh, H. C. (2015). Dynamin-related protein 1 mediates mitochondria-dependent apoptosis in chlorpyrifos-treated SH-SY5Y cells. *Neurotoxicology*, 51: 145–157. https://doi.org/10.1016/j.neuro.2015.10.008.

Pan, R. Y., Ma, J., Kong, X. X., Wang, X. F., Li, S. S., Qi, X. L., Yan, Y. H., Cheng, J., Liu, Q., Jin, W., Tan, C. H., and Yuan, Z. (2019). Sodium rutin ameliorates Alzheimer's disease-like pathology by enhancing microglial amyloid-β clearance. *Science advances*, 5(2): eaau6328. https://doi.org/10.1126/sciadv.aau6328.

Park, J. H., Zhuang, J., Li, J., and Hwang, P. M. (2016). p53 as guardian of the mitochondrial genome. *FEBS letters*, 590(7): 924–934. https://doi.org/10.1002/1873-3468.12061.

Park, J. S., Park, J. H., and Kim, K. Y. (2019). Neuroprotective effects of myristargenol A against glutamate-induced apoptotic HT22 cell death. *RSV Advances*, 9: 31247-31254. https://doi.org/10.1039/C9RA 05408A.

Paula, P. C., Angelica Maria, S. G., Luis, C. H., and Gloria Patricia, C. G. (2019). Preventive effect of quercetin in a triple transgenic Alzheimer's disease mice model. *Molecules (Basel, Switzerland)*, 24(12): 2287. https://doi.org/10.3390/molecules24122287.

Pehar, M., Ko, M. H., Li, M., Scrable, H., and Puglielli, L. (2014). P44, the 'longevity-assurance' isoform of P53, regulates tau phosphorylation and is activated in an age-dependent fashion. *Aging cell*, 13(3): 449–456. https://doi.org/10.1111/acel.12192.

Pervin, M., Unno, K., Ohishi, T., Tanabe, H., Miyoshi, N., and Nakamura, Y. (2018). Beneficial effects of green tea catechins on neurodegenerative diseases. *Molecules (Basel, Switzerland)*, 23(6): 1297. https://doi.org/10.3390/molecules23061297.

Phatak, V. M., and Muller, P. A. J. (2015). Metal toxicity and the p53 protein: an intimate relationship. *Toxicology research*, 4: 576-591. https://doi.org/10.1039/c4tx00117f.

Plesnila, N., von Baumgarten, L., Retiounskaia, M., Engel, D., Ardeshiri, A., Zimmermann, R., Hoffmann, F., Landshamer, S., Wagner, E., and Culmsee, C. (2007). Delayed neuronal death after brain trauma involves p53-dependent inhibition of NF-kappaB transcriptional activity. *Cell death and differentiation*, 14(8): 1529–1541. https://doi.org/10.1038/sj.cdd.4402159.

Puca, R., Nardinocchi, L., Sacchi, A., Rechavi, G., Givol, D., and D'Orazi, G. (2009). HIPK2 modulates p53 activity towards pro-apoptotic transcription. *Molecular cancer*, 8: 85. https://doi.org/10.1186/1476-4598-8-85.

Qin, J., Chen, H. G., Yan, Q., Deng, M., Liu, J., Doerge, S., Ma, W., Dong, Z., and Li, D. W. (2008). Protein phosphatase-2A is a target of epigallocatechin-3-gallate and modulates p53-Bak apoptotic pathway. *Cancer research*, 68(11): 4150–4162. https://doi.org/10.1158/0008-5472.CAN-08-0839.

Rachmany, L., Tweedie, D., Rubovitch, V., Yu, Q. S., Li, Y., Wang, J. Y., Pick, C. G., and Greig, N. H. (2013). Cognitive impairments accompanying rodent mild traumatic brain injury involve p53-dependent neuronal cell death and are ameliorated by the tetrahydrobenzothiazole PFT-α. *PloS one*, 8(11): e79837. https://doi.org/10.1371/journal.pone.0079837.

Radad, K., Moldzio, R., Taha, M., and Rausch, W. D. (2009). Thymoquinone protects dopaminergic neurons against MPP$^+$ and rotenone. *Phytotherapy research: PTR*, 23(5): 696–700. https://doi.org/10.1002/ptr.2708.

Radovanović, V., Vlainić, J., Hanžić, N., Ukić, P., Oršolić, N., Baranović, G., and Jazvinšćak Jembrek, M. (2019). Neurotoxic effect of ethanolic extract of propolis in the presence of copper ions is mediated through enhanced production of ROS and stimulation of caspase-3/7 activity. *Toxins*, 11(5): 273. https://doi.org/10.3390/toxins11050273.

Rane, J. S., Bhaumik, P., and Panda, D. (2017). Curcumin inhibits tau aggregation and disintegrates preformed tau filaments *in vitro*. *Journal of Alzheimer's disease: JAD*, 60(3): 999–1014. https://doi.org/10.3233/JAD-170351.

Raval, A. P., Dave, K. R., and Pérez-Pinzón, M. A. (2006). Resveratrol mimics ischemic preconditioning in the brain. *Journal of cerebral blood flow and metabolism: official journal of the International Society of Cerebral Blood Flow and Metabolism*, 26(9): 1141–1147. https://doi.org/10.1038/sj.jcbfm.9600262.

Reddy, P. H., Manczak, M., Yin, X., Grady, M. C., Mitchell, A., Tonk, S., Kuruva, C. S., Bhatti, J. S., Kandimalla, R., Vijayan, M., Kumar, S., Wang, R., Pradeepkiran, J. A., Ogunmokun, G., Thamarai, K., Quesada,

K., Boles, A., and Reddy, A. P. (2018). Protective effects of Indian spice curcumin against amyloid-β in Alzheimer's disease. *Journal of Alzheimer's disease: JAD*, 61(3): 843–866. https://doi.org/10.3233/JAD-170512.

Renaud, J., Bournival, J., Zottig, X., and Martinoli, M. G. (2014). Resveratrol protects DAergic PC12 cells from high glucose-induced oxidative stress and apoptosis: effect on p53 and GRP75 localization. *Neurotoxicity research*, 25(1): 110–123. https://doi.org/10.1007/s12640-013-9439-7.

Rezai-Zadeh, K., Arendash, G. W., Hou, H., Fernandez, F., Jensen, M., Runfeldt, M., Shytle, R. D., and Tan, J. (2008). Green tea epigallocatechin-3-gallate (EGCG) reduces beta-amyloid mediated cognitive impairment and modulates tau pathology in Alzheimer transgenic mice. *Brain research*, 1214: 177–187. https://doi.org/10.1016/j.brainres.2008.02.107.

Rishitha, N., and Muthuraman, A. (2018). Therapeutic evaluation of solid lipid nanoparticle of quercetin in pentylenetetrazole induced cognitive impairment of zebrafish. *Life sciences*, 199: 80–87. https://doi.org/10.1016/j.lfs.2018.03.010.

Rokavec, M., Li, H., Jiang, L., and Hermeking, H. (2014). The p53/miR-34 axis in development and disease. *Journal of molecular cell biology*, 6(3): 214–230. https://doi.org/10.1093/jmcb/mju003.

Sakhi, S., Sun, N., Wing, L. L., Mehta, P., and Schreiber, S. S. (1996). Nuclear accumulation of p53 protein following kainic acid-induced seizures. *Neuroreport*, 7(2): 493–496. https://doi.org/10.1097/00001756-199601310-00028.

Sandhir, R., and Mehrotra, A. (2013). Quercetin supplementation is effective in improving mitochondrial dysfunctions induced by 3-nitropropionic acid: implications in Huntington's disease. *Biochimica et biophysica acta*, 1832(3): 421–430. https://doi.org/10.1016/j.bbadis.2012.11.018.

Schroeder, E. K., Kelsey, N. A., Doyle, J., Breed, E., Bouchard, R. J., Loucks, F. A., Harbison, R. A., and Linseman, D. A. (2009). Green tea epigallocatechin 3-gallate accumulates in mitochondria and displays a selective antiapoptotic effect against inducers of mitochondrial oxidative stress in neurons. *Antioxidants & redox signaling*, 11(3): 469–480. https://doi.org/10.1089/ars.2008.2215.

Schuler, M. and Green, D. R. (2005). Transcription, apoptosis and p53: catch-22. *Trends in genetics: TIG*, 21(3): 182–187. https://doi.org/10.1016/j.tig.2005.01.001.

Shah, S. A., Lee, H. Y., Bressan, R. A., Yun, D. J., and Kim, M. O. (2014). Novel osmotin attenuates glutamate-induced synaptic dysfunction and neurodegeneration via the JNK/PI3K/Akt pathway in postnatal rat brain. *Cell death & disease*, 5(1), e1026. https://doi.org/10.1038/cddis.2013.538.

Sharma, D. R., Wani, W. Y., Sunkaria, A., Kandimalla, R. J., Sharma, R. K., Verma, D., Bal, A., and Gill, K. D. (2016). Quercetin attenuates neuronal death against aluminum-induced neurodegeneration in the rat hippocampus. *Neuroscience*, 324: 163–176. https://doi.org/10.1016/j.neuroscience.2016.02.055.

Sharma, N., and Nehru, B. (2018). Curcumin affords neuroprotection and inhibits α-synuclein aggregation in lipopolysaccharide-induced Parkinson's disease model. *Inflammopharmacology*, 26(2): 349–360. https://doi.org/10.1007/s10787-017-0402-8.

Shen, X. Y., Luo, T., Li, S., Ting, O. Y., He, F., Xu, J., and Wang, H. Q. (2018). Quercetin inhibits okadaic acid-induced tau protein hyperphosphorylation through the Ca^{2+}-calpain-p25-CDK5 pathway in HT22 cells. *International journal of molecular medicine*, 41(2): 1138–1146. https://doi.org/10.3892/ijmm.2017.3281

Shin, W. H., Park, S. J., and Kim, E. J. (2006). Protective effect of anthocyanins in middle cerebral artery occlusion and reperfusion model of cerebral ischemia in rats. *Life sciences*, 79(2): 130–137. https://doi.org/10.1016/j.lfs.2005.12.033.

Shytle, R. D., Tan, J., Bickford, P. C., Rezai-Zadeh, K., Hou, L., Zeng, J., Sanberg, P. R., Sanberg, C. D., Alberte, R. S., Fink, R. C., and Roschek, B., Jr (2012). Optimized turmeric extract reduces β-Amyloid and phosphorylated Tau protein burden in Alzheimer's transgenic mice. *Current Alzheimer research*, 9(4): 500–506. https://doi.org/10.2174/156720512800492459.

Šimić, G., Šešo-Šimić, Đ., Lucassen, P. J., Islam, A., Krsnik, Ž., Cviko, A., Jelašić, D., Barišić, N., Winblad, B., Kostović, I., and Krušlin, B. (2000a). Ultrastructural analysis and TUNEL demonstrate motor neuron apoptosis in Werdnig-Hoffmann disease. *The Journal of Neuropathology and Experimental Neurology*, 59(5): 398–407. https://doi.org/10.1093/jnen/59.5.398.

Šimić, G., Lucassen, P. J., Krsnik, Ž., Krušlin, B., Kostović, I., Winblad, B., and Bogdanović, N. (2000b). nNOS expression in reactive astrocytes correlates with increased cell death related DNA damage in the hippocampus and entorhinal cortex in Alzheimer's disease. *Experimental neurology*, 165(1): 12–26. https://doi.org/10.1006/exnr.2000.7448.

Šimić, G., Stanić, G., Mladinov, M., Jovanov Milošević, N., Kostović, I., and Hof, P. R. (2009) Does Alzheimer's disease begin in the brainstem? *Neuropathology and Applied Neurobiology*, 35(6): 532-554. https://doi.org/10.1111/j.1365-2990.2009.01038.x.

Šimić, G., Babić Leko, M., Wray, S., Harrington, C., Delalle, I., Jovanov-Milošević, N., Bažadona, D., Buée, L., de Silva, R., Di Giovanni, G., Wischik, C., and Hof, P. R. (2016) Tau protein hyperphosphorylation and aggregation in Alzheimer's disease and other tauopathies, and possible neuroprotective strategies. *Biomolecules*, 2016 (6): E6. https://doi.org/10.3390/biom6010006

Šimić, G., Španić, E., Langer Horvat, L., and Hof, P. R. (2019) Blood-brain barrier and innate immunity in the pathogenesis of Alzheimer's disease. *Progress in Molecular Biology and Translational Science*, 168: 99-145. https://doi.org/10.1016/bs.pmbts.2019.06.003.

Singh, N. A., Mandal, A. K., and Khan, Z. A. (2016). Potential neuroprotective properties of epigallocatechin-3-gallate (EGCG). *Nutrition journal*, 15(1): 60. https://doi.org/10.1186/s12937-016-0179-4.

Španić, E., Langer Horvat, L., Hof, P. R., and Šimić, G. (2019) Role of microglial cells in Alzheimer's disease tau propagation. *Frontiers in Aging Neuroscience*, 11:271. https://doi.org/10.3389/fnagi.2019.00271.

Speidel D. (2010). Transcription-independent p53 apoptosis: an alternative route to death. *Trends in cell biology*, 20(1): 14–24. https://doi.org/10.1016/j.tcb.2009.10.002.

Stanga, S., Lanni, C., Govoni, S., Uberti, D., D'Orazi, G., and Racchi, M. (2010). Unfolded p53 in the pathogenesis of Alzheimer's disease: is HIPK2 the link? *Aging*, 2(9): 545–554. https://doi.org/10.18632/aging.100205.

Steckley, D., Karajgikar, M., Dale, L. B., Fuerth, B., Swan, P., Drummond-Main, C., Poulter, M. O., Ferguson, S. S., Strasser, A., and Cregan, S. P. (2007). Puma is a dominant regulator of oxidative stress induced Bax activation and neuronal apoptosis. *The Journal of neuroscience: the official journal of the Society for Neuroscience*, 27(47): 12989–12999. https://doi.org/10.1523/JNEUROSCI.3400-07.2007.

Strathearn, K. E., Yousef, G. G., Grace, M. H., Roy, S. L., Tambe, M. A., Ferruzzi, M. G., Wu, Q. L., Simon, J. E., Lila, M. A., and Rochet, J. C. (2014). Neuroprotective effects of anthocyanin- and proanthocyanidin-rich extracts in cellular models of Parkinson's disease. *Brain research*, 1555: 60–77. https://doi.org/10.1016/j.brainres.2014.01.047.

Su, B., Wang, X., Lee, H. G., Tabaton, M., Perry, G., Smith, M. A., and Zhu, X. (2010). Chronic oxidative stress causes increased tau phosphorylation in M17 neuroblastoma cells. *Neuroscience letters*, 468(3): 267–271. https://doi.org/10.1016/j.neulet.2009.11.010.

Sullivan, K. D., Galbraith, M. D., Andrysik, Z., and Espinosa, J. M. (2018). Mechanisms of transcriptional regulation by p53. *Cell death and differentiation*, 25(1): 133–143. https://doi.org/10.1038/cdd.2017.174.

Szybińska, A., and Leśniak, W. (2017). P53 dysfunction in neurodegenerative diseases - the cause or effect of pathological changes?. *Aging and disease*, 8(4): 506–518. https://doi.org/10.14336/AD.2016.1120.

Tan, X., Yang, Y., Xu, J., Zhang, P., Deng, R., Mao, Y., He, J., Chen, Y., Zhang, Y., Ding, J., Li, H., Shen, H., Li, X., Dong, W., and Chen, G. (2020a). Luteolin exerts neuroprotection *via* modulation of the p62/Keap1/Nrf2 Pathway in intracerebral hemorrhage. *Frontiers in pharmacology*, 10: 1551. https://doi.org/10.3389/fphar.2019.01551.

Tan, X. H., Zhang, K. K., Xu, J. T., Qu, D., Chen, L. J., Li, J. H., Wang, Q., Wang, H. J., and Xie, X. L. (2020b). Luteolin alleviates methamphetamine-induced neurotoxicity by suppressing PI3K/Akt pathway-modulated apoptosis and autophagy in rats. *Food and chemical toxicology: an international journal published for the British Industrial Biological Research Association*, 137: 111179. https://doi.org/10.1016/j.fct.2020.111179.

Teng, Y., Zhao, J., Ding, L., Ding, Y., and Zhou, P. (2019). Complex of EGCG with Cu(II) suppresses amyloid aggregation and Cu(II)-induced cytotoxicity of α-synuclein. *Molecules (Basel, Switzerland)*, 24(16): 2940. https://doi.org/10.3390/molecules24162940.

Turnquist, C., Horikawa, I., Foran, E., Major, E. O., Vojtesek, B., Lane, D. P., Lu, X., Harris, B. T., and Harris, C. C. (2016). p53 isoforms regulate astrocyte-mediated neuroprotection and neurodegeneration. *Cell death and differentiation*, 23(9): 1515–1528. https://doi.org/10.1038/cdd.2016.37.

Uddin, M. S., and Kabir, M. T. (2019). Emerging signal regulating potential of genistein against Alzheimer's disease: a promising molecule of interest. *Frontiers in cell and developmental biology*, 7: 197. https://doi.org/10.3389/fcell.2019.00197.

Uo, T., Veenstra, T. D., and Morrison, R. S. (2009). Histone deacetylase inhibitors prevent p53-dependent and p53-independent Bax-mediated neuronal apoptosis through two distinct mechanisms. *The Journal of neuroscience: the official journal of the Society for Neuroscience*, 29(9): 2824–2832. https://doi.org/10.1523/JNEUROSCI.6186-08.2009.

van Dieck, J., Fernandez-Fernandez, M. R., Veprintsev, D. B., and Fersht, A. R. (2009). Modulation of the oligomerization state of p53 by differential binding of proteins of the S100 family to p53 monomers and tetramers. *The Journal of biological chemistry*, 284(20): 13804–13811. https://doi.org/10.1074/jbc.M901351200.

Vaseva, A. V., Marchenko, N. D., Ji, K., Tsirka, S. E., Holzmann, S., and Moll, U. M. (2012). p53 opens the mitochondrial permeability transition pore to trigger necrosis. *Cell*, 149(7): 1536–1548. https://doi.org/10.1016/j.cell.2012.05.014.

Vauzour, D., Vafeiadou, K., Rodriguez-Mateos, A., Rendeiro, C., and Spencer, J. P. (2008). The neuroprotective potential of flavonoids: a multiplicity of effects. *Genes & nutrition*, 3(3-4): 115–126. https://doi.org/10.1007/s12263-008-0091-4.

Velazhahan, V., Glaza, P., Herrera, A. I., Prakash, O., Zolkiewski, M., Geisbrecht, B. V., and Schrick, K. (2020). Dietary flavonoid fisetin binds human SUMO1 and blocks sumoylation of p53. *PloS one*, 15(6): e0234468. https://doi.org/10.1371/journal.pone.0234468.

Vieler, M., and Sanyal, S. (2018). p53 isoforms and their implications in cancer. *Cancers*, 10(9): 288. https://doi.org/10.3390/cancers10090288.

Wang, C. M., Liu, M. Y., Wang, F., Wei, M. J., Wang, S., Wu, C. F., and Yang, J. Y. (2013). Anti-amnesic effect of pseudoginsenoside-F11 in two mouse models of Alzheimer's disease. *Pharmacology, biochemistry, and behavior*, 106: 57–67. https://doi.org/10.1016/j.pbb.2013.03.010.

Wang, D. B., Kinoshita, C., Kinoshita, Y., and Morrison, R. S. (2014). p53 and mitochondrial function in neurons. *Biochimica et biophysica acta*, 1842(8): 1186–1197. https://doi.org/10.1016/j.bbadis.2013.12.015.

Wang, L., He, G., Zhang, P., Wang, X., Jiang, M., and Yu, L. (2011). Interplay between MDM2, MDMX, Pirh2 and COP1: the negative regulators of p53. *Molecular biology reports*, 38(1): 229–236. https://doi.org/10.1007/s11033-010-0099-x.

Wang, H., Xu, Y. S., Wang, M. L., Cheng, C., Bian, R., Yuan, H., Wang, Y., Guo, T., Zhu, L. L., and Zhou, H. (2017). Protective effect of naringin against the LPS-induced apoptosis of PC12 cells: Implications for the treatment of neurodegenerative disorders. *International journal of molecular medicine*, 39(4): 819–830. https://doi.org/10.3892/ijmm.2017.2904.

Wang, Y., Dong, X. X., Cao, Y., Liang, Z. Q., Han, R., Wu, J. C., Gu, Z. L., and Qin, Z. H. (2009). p53 induction contributes to excitotoxic neuronal death in rat striatum through apoptotic and autophagic mechanisms. *The*

European journal of neuroscience, 30(12): 2258–2270. https://doi.org/10.1111/j.1460-9568.2009.07025.x.

Wanninger, S., Lorenz, V., Subhan, A., and Edelmann, F. T. (2015). Metal complexes of curcumin--synthetic strategies, structures and medicinal applications. *Chemical Society reviews*, 44(15): 4986–5002. https://doi.org/10.1039/c5cs00088b.

Wei, J., Zaika, E., and Zaika, A. (2012). p53 family: role of protein isoforms in human cancer. *Journal of nucleic acids*, 2012: 687359. https://doi.org/10.1155/2012/687359.

Wei, J., Zhang, G., Zhang, X., Xu, D., Gao, J., Fan, J., and Zhou, Z. (2017). Anthocyanins from Black Chokeberry (Aroniamelanocarpa Elliot) Delayed Aging-Related Degenerative Changes of Brain. *Journal of agricultural and food chemistry*, 65(29): 5973–5984. https://doi.org/10.1021/acs.jafc.7b02136.

Wobst, H. J., Sharma, A., Diamond, M. I., Wanker, E. E., and Bieschke, J. (2015). The green tea polyphenol (-)-epigallocatechin gallate prevents the aggregation of tau protein into toxic oligomers at substoichiometric ratios. *FEBS letters*, 589(1): 77–83. https://doi.org/10.1016/j.febslet.2014.11.026.

Wu, S. Y., and Chiang, C. M. (2009). Crosstalk between sumoylation and acetylation regulates p53-dependent chromatin transcription and DNA binding. *The EMBO journal*, 28(9): 1246–1259. https://doi.org/10.1038/emboj.2009.83.

Yakovlev, V. A., Bayden, A. S., Graves, P. R., Kellogg, G. E., and Mikkelsen, R. B. (2010). Nitration of the tumor suppressor protein p53 at tyrosine 327 promotes p53 oligomerization and activation. *Biochemistry*, 49(25): 5331–5339. https://doi.org/10.1021/bi100564w.

Yamauchi, R., Sasaki, K., and Yoshida, K. (2009). Identification of epigallocatechin-3-gallate in green tea polyphenols as a potent inducer of p53-dependent apoptosis in the human lung cancer cell line A549. *Toxicology in vitro: an international journal published in association with BIBRA*, 23(5): 834–839. https://doi.org/10.1016/j.tiv.2009.04.011.

Yang, X., Si, P., Qin, H., Yin, L., Yan, L. J., & Zhang, C. (2017). The neuroprotective effects of SIRT1 on NMDA-induced excitotoxicity.

Oxidative medicine and cellular longevity, 2017: 2823454. https://doi.org/10.1155/2017/2823454.

Yousef, M. I., Khalil, D., and Abdou, H. M. (2018). Neuro- and nephroprotective effect of grape seed proanthocyanidin extract against carboplatin and thalidomide through modulation of inflammation, tumor suppressor protein p53, neurotransmitters, oxidative stress and histology. *Toxicology reports*, 5: 568–578. https://doi.org/10.1016/j.toxrep.2018.04.006.

Yu, H. L., Li, L., Zhang, X. H., Xiang, L., Zhang, J., Feng, J. F., and Xiao, R. (2009). Neuroprotective effects of genistein and folic acid on apoptosis of rat cultured cortical neurons induced by beta-amyloid 31-35. *The British journal of nutrition*, 102(5): 655–662. https://doi.org/10.1017/S0007114509243042.

Yu, C., Zhang, P., Lou, L., and Wang, Y. (2019). Perspectives regarding the role of biochanin A in humans. *Frontiers in pharmacology*, 10: 793. https://doi.org/10.3389/fphar.2019.00793.

Xu, Q., Chen, Z., Zhu, B., Wang, G., Jia, Q., Li, Y., and Wu, X. (2020). A-type cinnamon procyanidin oligomers protect against 1-methyl-4-phenyl-1,2,3,6-tetrahydropyridine-induced neurotoxicity in mice through inhibiting the p38 mitogen-activated protein kinase/p53/BCL-2 associated X protein signaling pathway. *The Journal of nutrition*, 150(7): 1731–1737. https://doi.org/10.1093/jn/nxaa128.

Zeng, K. W., Liao, L. X., Zhao, M. B., Song, F. J., Yu, Q., Jiang, Y., and Tu, P. F. (2015). Protosappanin B protects PC12 cells against oxygen-glucose deprivation-induced neuronal death by maintaining mitochondrial homeostasis via induction of ubiquitin-dependent p53 protein degradation. *European journal of pharmacology*, 751: 13–23. https://doi.org/10.1016/j.ejphar.2015.01.039.

Zhang, F., Peng, W., Zhang, J., Dong, W., Wu, J., Wang, T., and Xie, Z. (2020). P53 and Parkin co-regulate mitophagy in bone marrow mesenchymal stem cells to promote the repair of early steroid-induced osteonecrosis of the femoral head. *Cell death & disease*, 11(1): 42. https://doi.org/10.1038/s41419-020-2238-1.

Zhao, H., Liang, J., Li, X., Yu, H., Li, X., and Xiao, R. (2010). Folic acid and soybean isoflavone combined supplementation protects the post-neural tube closure defects of rodents induced by cyclophosphamide *in vivo* and *in vitro*. *Neurotoxicology*, 31(2): 180–187. https://doi.org/10.1016/j.neuro.2009.12.011.

Zhao, L. P., Ji, C., Lu, P. H., Li, C., Xu, B., and Gao, H. (2013a). Oxygen glucose deprivation (OGD)/re-oxygenation-induced *in vitro* neuronal cell death involves mitochondrial cyclophilin-D/P53 signaling axis. *Neurochemical research*, 38(4): 705–713. https://doi.org/10.1007/s11064-013-0968-5.

Zhao, L., Wang, J. L., Wang, Y. R., and Fa, X. Z. (2013b). Apigenin attenuates copper-mediated β-amyloid neurotoxicity through antioxidation, mitochondrion protection and MAPK signal inactivation in an AD cell model. *Brain research*, 1492: 33–45. https://doi.org/10.1016/j.brainres.2012.11.019.

Zhou, F., Chen, S., Xiong, J., Li, Y., and Qu, L. (2012). Luteolin reduces zinc-induced tau phosphorylation at Ser262/356 in an ROS-dependent manner in SH-SY5Y cells. *Biological trace element research*, 149(2): 273–279. https://doi.org/10.1007/s12011-012-9411-z.

Zhou, F., Qu, L., Lv, K., Chen, H., Liu, J., Liu, X., Li, Y., and Sun, X. (2011). Luteolin protects against reactive oxygen species-mediated cell death induced by zinc toxicity via the PI3K-Akt-NF-κB-ERK-dependent pathway. *Journal of neuroscience research*, 89(11): 1859–1868. https://doi.org/10.1002/jnr.22714.

Zhou, L. J., and Zhu, X. Z. (2000). Reactive oxygen species-induced apoptosis in PC12 cells and protective effect of bilobalide. *The Journal of pharmacology and experimental therapeutics*, 293(3): 982–988.

Zhu, G., Wang, X., Wu, S., and Li, Q. (2012). Involvement of activation of PI3K/Akt pathway in the protective effects of puerarin against MPP+-induced human neuroblastoma SH-SY5Y cell death. *Neurochemistry international*, 60(4): 400–408. https://doi.org/10.1016/j.neuint.2012.01.003.

Zhu, J., Mu, X., Zeng, J., Xu, C., Liu, J., Zhang, M., Li, C., Chen, J., Li, T., and Wang, Y. (2014). Ginsenoside Rg1 prevents cognitive impairment and hippocampus senescence in a rat model of D-galactose-induced aging. *PloS one*, 9(6), e101291. https://doi.org/10.1371/journal.pone.0101291.

Zubčić, K., Radovanović, V., Vlainić, J., Hof, P. R., Oršolić, N., Šimić, G., and Jazvinšćak Jembrek, M. (2020). PI3K/Akt and ERK1/2 signalling are involved in quercetin-mediated neuroprotection against copper-induced injury. *Oxidative medicine and cellular longevity*, 2020: 9834742. https://doi.org/10.1155/2020/9834742.

INDEX

A

aberration, vii, 1, 2, 9, 12, 16, 23, 24, 25, 27, 28, 33, 34
acetylation, 3, 37, 131, 133, 148, 150, 153, 159, 178
acetylcholinesterase, 142, 152
acid, 129, 134, 142, 145, 165, 169, 172, 173, 180
active compound, 149
acute leukemia, 81
acute lymphoblastic leukemia, 7, 46, 47, 55, 56, 57, 65, 67, 70, 75, 79
acute lymphoblastic leukemia/lymphoma (ALL), iv, 7, 18, 20, 21, 22, 23, 24, 28, 31, 41, 72, 87, 106, 136
acute myelogenous leukemia, 50, 67
acute myeloid leukemia (AML), vii, 1, 4, 7, 8, 9, 10, 11, 12, 14, 15, 16, 17, 18, 19, 20, 22, 31, 43, 47, 48, 49, 50, 51, 53, 55, 56, 59, 61, 63, 64, 65, 66, 67, 68, 70, 71, 72, 77, 79, 81, 88, 89, 92, 99, 113, 114, 115
acute promyelocytic leukemia, 99

acute stress, 133
adaptive immunity, 8
adult T-cell leukemia (ATLL), 31, 34, 53, 71
aggregation, 142, 147, 151, 159, 165, 167, 171, 173, 174, 176, 178
allele, 9, 10, 15, 21, 62, 69, 86, 87, 89, 91, 92, 100
amyloid beta, 154, 156, 157
amyotrophic lateral sclerosis, 128, 148, 164
anaplastic large cell lymphoma (ALCL), 33, 34, 48
anaplastic T-cell lymphoma, 31
apoptosis, 2, 3, 4, 7, 12, 19, 22, 23, 30, 31, 32, 36, 37, 38, 39, 40, 44, 45, 49, 53, 55, 56, 61, 63, 68, 73, 84, 87, 88, 98, 99, 104, 121, 124, 129, 130, 132, 133, 134, 138, 141, 143, 144, 146, 147, 150, 151, 152, 153, 155, 156, 157, 158, 159, 160, 161, 162, 163,169, 172, 173, 174, 175, 176, 177, 178, 179, 180
apoptotic mechanisms, 141
apoptotic pathways, 31

arrest, 2, 3, 4, 19, 30, 31, 32, 49, 84, 87, 100, 159
arsenic, 122
arsenic trioxide (ATO), 99, 122

B

B-cell prolymphocytic leukemia (B-PLL), 23, 27, 45
behavioral change, 142
beneficial effect, 136, 147, 151
biliverdin reductase, 155
bioavailability, 153
biochemistry, 163, 164, 165, 177
biological activity, 143
blood, 7, 8, 42, 43, 44, 45, 47, 49, 50, 52, 54, 55, 56, 57, 60, 63, 64, 65, 67, 68, 69, 70, 71, 72, 74, 75, 77, 78, 79, 112, 113, 114, 140, 144
blood flow, 140
blood-brain barrier, 144
bone, 14, 19, 25, 32, 57, 82, 179
bone marrow, 14, 19, 25, 32, 57, 82, 179
brain, 132, 133, 134, 135, 138, 142, 143, 146, 155, 156, 157, 160, 165, 170, 171, 173, 174
Burkitt lymphoma (BL), 21, 23, 24, 28, 31, 51, 59, 60, 63

C

cancer, v, viii, 4, 7, 21, 36, 42, 43, 44, 45, 46, 47, 49, 50, 54, 55, 56, 58, 59, 61, 62, 64, 65, 67, 68, 69, 71, 73, 77, 79, 83, 84, 85, 86, 88, 89, 93, 95, 96, 97, 98, 99, 100, 101, 103, 104, 105, 106, 107, 108, 109, 110, 111, 115, 116, 117, 118, 119, 120, 121, 122, 123, 124, 125, 126, 144, 145, 154, 155, 163, 164, 166, 168, 171, 177, 178
cancer cells, viii, 83, 98, 100, 145
cancer progression, 101
cell biology, 161, 172, 175
cell cycle, 2, 3, 4, 19, 26, 29, 30, 31, 32, 49, 62, 79, 84, 87, 88, 109, 110, 122, 125, 155, 159, 164, 165, 166
cell cycle arrest, 2, 3, 4, 19, 30, 31, 32, 49, 84, 87
cell death, 3, 22, 74, 100, 138, 140, 152, 163, 167, 168, 170, 171, 174, 180
cell differentiation, 169
cell fate, 53, 153, 159, 160
cell line, 4, 11, 12, 13, 19, 22, 23, 31, 32, 36, 39, 40, 59, 162, 178
cellular homeostasis, 129
central nervous system, 154, 156, 158
cerebral blood flow, 171
cerebral cortex, 134
cetuximab, 100, 124
chemotherapy, 7, 8, 20, 22, 27, 31, 36, 48, 88, 93, 96, 97, 100
childhood, 55, 56, 57, 75, 79
chromosomal abnormalities, 9, 37
chromosomal alterations, 61
chromosome, 2, 13, 24, 42, 57, 81, 84, 91, 92
chromosome 17, 2, 13, 61, 84, 91, 92, 114
chronic lymphocytic leukemia, 7, 25, 43, 46, 48, 50, 51, 55, 56, 67, 78, 90
chronic lymphocytic leukemia (CLL), 7, 22, 24, 25, 31, 32, 43, 46, 48, 50, 51, 53, 55, 56, 58, 63, 67, 72, 78, 90
chronic lymphocytic leukemia/small lymphocytic lymphoma (CLL/SLL), 7, 24, 25, 31, 32
cleavage, 141, 146, 148, 150
clinical application, 143, 167
clinical symptoms, 136
clinical trials, 17, 41, 88, 99, 100
clonal hematopoiesis (CH), 7, 8, 9, 122
cognitive abilities, 143, 151
cognitive capacity, 149
cognitive function, 141, 146, 149

cognitive impairment, 134, 143, 146, 148, 150, 156, 160, 162, 172, 181
cognitive performance, 142
combination therapy, 17, 99
compounds, 32, 147, 152, 168
copper, 136, 141, 143, 145, 163, 171, 180, 181
correlation, 27, 46, 92, 97, 135
cortex, 134, 150, 151
cortical neurons, 132, 134, 145, 147, 148, 149, 150, 156, 165, 179
crizotinib, 96, 117
curcumin, 151, 153, 156, 158, 172, 178
cytotoxicity, 22, 30, 155, 176

DNA damage, 2, 3, 4, 6, 7, 84, 87, 89, 100, 102, 107, 125, 129, 131, 133, 135, 143, 147, 159, 167, 169, 174
DNA repair, 2, 5, 78, 84, 87, 139
dominant negative, vii, viii, 83, 84, 86, 87, 88, 106
dominant negative effect (DNE), vii, viii, 83, 84, 86, 87, 106
dopaminergic, 146, 148, 152, 162, 169, 171
down-regulation, viii, 1, 38, 160
dysfunction, vii, viii, 2, 29, 60, 66, 134, 139, 156, 157, 161, 164, 165, 168, 173, 175
dysregulation, vii, 1, 2, 11, 13, 29, 41, 50, 74, 136

D

defence, 136, 140, 143, 153
degradation, 2, 11, 18, 24, 26, 29, 38, 39, 41, 84, 98, 99, 131, 139, 145, 150, 179
deletion, 5, 7, 11, 13, 20, 21, 23, 24, 27, 28, 29, 33, 34, 35, 37, 41, 47, 48, 49, 50, 52, 53, 58, 60, 61, 63, 67, 71, 115
dementia, 149, 162, 164
deprivation, 2, 6, 133, 144, 148, 150, 179, 180
deregulation, 16, 33, 41, 44, 62
derivatives, 151, 153, 158, 169
diffuse large B-cell lymphoma (DLBCL), 23, 24, 28, 29, 30, 42, 47, 48, 54, 59, 60, 61, 73, 75, 76, 78, 79
disease model, 173
disease progression, vii, 1, 2, 24, 25, 35, 41, 55, 63
diseases, 64, 92, 153, 154, 155
DNA, 2, 3, 4, 5, 6, 7, 9, 11, 21, 23, 29, 32, 40, 64, 78, 84, 85, 87, 89, 92, 99, 100, 102, 104, 105, 107, 109, 120, 122, 125, 129, 130, 131, 132, 133, 134, 135, 136, 139, 143, 147, 148, 151, 157, 159, 163, 167, 169, 174, 178

E

E3 ligase, 29, 56, 84, 99, 122
E3 ubiquitin ligase, 2, 4, 38, 131, 139
E4 ubiquitin ligase, 84
encoding, viii, 27, 33, 83, 92
endogenous mechanisms, 136, 143
endometrial cancer, 99, 122
endothelial cells, 128, 152, 169
entorhinal cortex, 135, 174
environment, 132, 138, 153
environmental stress, 8
enzymes, 39, 137, 138, 141, 144, 147, 149, 150, 151
epigenetic modification, 9
epithelial ovarian cancer, 96
evidence, 8, 36, 68, 88, 89, 98, 100, 133
excitotoxicity, 134, 145, 151, 161, 169, 178
exons, 5, 6, 9, 23, 29
exposure, 100, 133, 141, 150, 151, 157
extracts, 146, 167, 175
extranodal marginal zone cell lymphoma with mucosa-associated lymphoid tissue (MALT), 23

F

flavonoids, viii, 128, 141, 143, 144, 145, 146, 147, 153, 167, 177
follicular lymphoma (FL), 24, 26, 44, 47, 57, 63, 64, 65
formation, 5, 40, 87, 135, 142, 149, 152, 168
functional analysis, 66
fusion, 11, 22, 46, 59, 85, 139

G

gain of function (GOF), vii, viii, 9, 37, 83, 86, 88, 89, 93, 98, 99, 100, 121
gene amplification, 24
gene expression, 4, 59, 68, 142, 148
genes, viii, 3, 5, 6, 13, 21, 22, 26, 28, 33, 35, 37, 42, 46, 49, 56, 57, 64, 75, 77, 78, 84, 85, 87, 89, 92, 96, 127, 130, 136, 137, 138, 142, 144, 153, 162, 166, 168
genetic alteration, 24, 57
genetic mutations, 9
genome, 2, 78, 86, 87, 93, 129, 139, 170
genome integrity, 86, 87
genomic instability, 86, 87, 88
glucose, 133, 140, 144, 148, 150, 172, 179, 180
glutamate, 133, 151, 170, 173
glutathione, 128, 137, 142, 145, 149, 152, 163
glycogen, 128, 137
glycolysis, 3, 4, 129, 138, 140
glycoside, 144
growth, 5, 7, 19, 25, 30, 32, 38, 39, 68, 99, 100, 131, 159
growth arrest, 131
growth factor, 100
guardian, 2, 129, 170

H

hallmarks of cancer, 86
head and neck cancers, 97
health, 139, 141, 151, 153, 160
health effects, 152
hemaologic maligancies, 89
hematologic neoplasms, vii, viii, 1, 2, 41
hippocampus, 134, 142, 143, 146, 148, 149, 150, 151, 154, 164, 173, 174, 181
histone, 37, 38, 99, 133
histone deacetylase, 38, 99, 133
histone deacetylase 6 (HDAC6), 99, 121
homeostasis, 73, 130, 136, 139, 146, 147, 150, 163, 179
human, vii, viii, 1, 2, 5, 13, 17, 19, 34, 44, 49, 51, 56, 58, 59, 66, 76, 81, 83, 84, 93, 96, 100, 128, 132, 135, 149, 152, 153, 161, 163, 167, 169, 177, 178, 180
human health, 153
hydrogen, 128, 134, 141, 161, 163
hydrogen bonds, 141
hydrogen peroxide, 128, 134, 161, 163
hypermethylation, 37
hypoxia, 2, 6

I

immunohistochemistry, 93, 96, 97
immunohistochemistry (IHC), 93, 96, 97
immunoreactivity, 97, 134
in vitro, vii, ix, 13, 19, 22, 23, 41, 68, 81, 88, 98, 99, 128, 143, 146, 171, 178, 180
in vivo, vii, ix, 19, 22, 39, 41, 68, 98, 128, 158, 180
incidence, vii, 1, 8, 10, 12, 20, 21, 23, 24, 34, 35, 41, 57, 61, 64
induction, 7, 15, 19, 27, 30, 31, 32, 38, 39, 40, 44, 46, 68, 69, 98, 99, 133, 134, 145, 148, 177, 179

inflammation, 8, 136, 143, 145, 155, 159, 179
inhibition, 2, 19, 22, 37, 38, 39, 40, 45, 46, 88, 98, 100, 101, 133, 164, 168, 170
inhibitor, 17, 18, 19, 22, 31, 37, 38, 39, 40, 41, 44, 45, 48, 50, 51, 54, 55, 56, 60, 61, 66, 68, 72, 76, 96, 99, 100, 121, 133, 144, 149, 157, 165
injury, iv, 131, 132, 133, 134, 138, 143, 144, 146, 148, 151, 160, 163, 166, 169, 181
innate immunity, 13, 174
integrity, 2, 84, 86, 87, 139
intracerebral hemorrhage, 176
ischemia, 133, 143, 148, 159, 164, 173
ischemia-reperfusion injury, 159

K

karyotype, vii, 1, 9, 11, 13, 59, 68, 92

L

landscape, 43, 60, 101, 154
leukemia, 11, 17, 20, 22, 23, 24, 27, 31, 34, 35, 45, 47, 53, 54, 56, 63, 71, 74, 81, 82
lipid metabolism, 140
lipid peroxidation, 138, 141, 143, 144, 147, 149, 150
localization, 5, 6, 135, 172
locus, 7, 11, 29, 37, 50, 84
longevity, 154, 157, 160, 162, 167, 170, 179, 181
loss of function, vii, viii, 83, 84, 87, 88
loss of heterozygosity (LOH), 87, 88, 92
lung cancer, 93, 95, 100, 104, 111, 115, 116, 117, 178
lymphoblastic leukemia/lymphoma (ALL), iv, 7, 18, 20, 21, 22, 23, 24, 28, 31, 41, 72, 87, 106, 136
lymphoid, vii, 1, 23, 25, 46, 51, 75

lymphoid tissue, vii, 1, 23
lymphoma, vii, 1, 7, 20, 21, 23, 24, 25, 26, 27, 28, 29, 30, 31, 33, 34, 42, 43, 44, 47, 48, 49, 50, 51, 52, 53, 54, 55, 59, 60, 61, 62, 63, 64, 65, 66, 69, 70, 72, 73, 75, 76, 78, 79, 82

M

malignancy, 7, 9, 34, 35, 52
management, 66, 149, 153, 169
manganese, 138, 155
mantle, 23, 50, 52, 53, 54, 55, 69, 70, 72, 73
mantle cell lymphoma (MCL), 23, 24, 27, 31, 32, 38, 50, 52, 53, 54, 55, 69, 70, 72, 73
median, 13, 16, 21, 26, 27, 29, 30, 35, 36
medicine, 154, 157, 159, 160, 162, 163, 166, 167, 169, 179, 181
memory, 142, 146, 151, 154, 164
memory function, 146, 164
mesenchymal stem cells, 179
metabolic pathways, 101
metabolism, 3, 86, 139, 141, 166, 168, 171
metal ion, 140, 152, 163
metastasis, viii, 4, 83, 86, 88, 100
methamphetamine, 145, 176
methylation, 3, 11, 30, 37, 41, 42, 64, 131
mice, 13, 23, 32, 37, 40, 134, 136, 138, 142, 143, 145, 146, 148, 150, 151, 152, 156, 159, 164, 170, 172, 173, 179
microRNA, viii, 1, 53, 59, 62, 77
microRNA (miRNA), viii, 1, 4, 9, 12, 16, 36, 37, 53, 59, 62, 68, 77
microscopy, 163
midbrain, 146, 148, 152, 169
migration, 38, 40, 86
MIRA-1, 40, 41, 68
mitochondria, 132, 138, 139, 143, 169, 172
mitochondrial damage, 139, 160
mitochondrial DNA, 129, 139

mitogen, 128, 137, 179
models, vii, ix, 8, 23, 31, 67, 88, 98, 128, 136, 139, 143, 146, 149, 151, 153, 164, 175, 177
modifications, viii, 3, 84, 127, 131, 153, 159
molecular medicine, 163, 173, 177
molecular structure, 146
molecular weight, 32
molecules, 16, 30, 40, 41, 69, 167, 169
mRNA, 4, 11, 12, 19, 36, 37, 59, 149
multiple myeloma (MM), vii, 1, 4, 7, 32, 35, 36, 37, 38, 39, 40, 41, 42, 43, 45, 47, 48, 49, 50, 51, 52, 53, 54, 58, 59, 60, 62, 65, 66, 67, 68, 69, 73, 74, 79, 99, 122
murine double minute 2 (MDM2), viii, 1, 2, 3, 4, 6, 11, 13, 16, 17, 18, 19, 22, 24, 26, 28, 29, 30, 31, 33, 36, 37, 38, 39, 41, 42, 44, 45, 46, 48, 49, 50, 51, 53, 54, 55, 56, 61, 62, 65, 67, 68, 70, 72, 73, 74, 75, 78, 79, 84, 98, 99, 102, 106, 120, 121, 128, 131, 144, 177
murine double minute 4 (MDM4), 2, 3, 4, 6, 11, 16, 19, 22, 26, 28, 29, 30, 39, 41, 53, 59, 131, 167
mutant, viii, 4, 8, 9, 11, 15, 18, 19, 20, 23, 28, 30, 32, 40, 41, 44, 47, 70, 77, 79, 83, 84, 85, 86, 87, 88, 89, 92, 93, 95, 97, 98, 99, 100, 101, 121, 145, 148
mutation, v, viii, 1, 5, 8, 9, 10, 11, 12, 13, 14, 15, 16, 20, 21, 23, 24, 26, 27, 28, 29, 30, 33, 34, 35, 36, 42, 46, 47, 53, 61, 63, 64, 69, 71, 83, 85, 88, 89, 90, 91, 92, 93, 94, 95, 96, 97, 99, 103, 106, 107, 116, 117, 118, 119, 122
mutational analysis, 66, 97
mutations, vii, viii, 5, 6, 7, 8, 9, 10, 12, 13, 14, 15, 16, 20, 21, 23, 25, 26, 27, 28, 29, 31, 32, 34, 35, 36, 41, 43, 46, 48, 50, 51, 52, 54, 55, 57, 59, 60, 64, 65, 66, 67, 69, 72, 73, 75, 78, 83, 84, 85, 86, 87, 88, 89, 91, 92, 93, 94, 95, 96, 97, 99, 139
mycosis fungoides (MF), 34

myelodysplastic syndromes, 52, 53, 55, 58, 60, 61, 62, 64, 66, 68, 69, 72, 73, 79
myelodysplatic dysplastic syndromes (MDS), 7, 10, 12, 13, 14, 15, 16, 17, 19, 20, 47, 62, 63, 70, 72, 89, 91, 92
myeloproliferative neoplasms (MPN), 15, 60, 66, 73

N

natural compound, vii, ix, 128, 140, 153
neurobiology, 157, 162, 164, 165
neuroblastoma, 132, 149, 150, 158, 167, 175, 180
neurodegeneration, ix, 128, 134, 136, 139, 140, 142, 143, 147, 153, 154, 156, 164, 168, 173, 176
neurodegenerative diseases, vii, viii, ix, 127, 128, 130, 140, 141, 153, 155, 156, 157, 160, 165, 167, 168, 170, 175
neurodegenerative disorders, 177
neurogenesis, 147, 149, 151
neuroinflammation, 140, 143, 147, 161, 162
neuronal apoptosis, 132, 134, 141, 147, 150, 151, 153, 159, 162, 175, 176
neuronal cells, 132, 135, 140, 161
neurons, viii, 127, 132, 133, 137, 138, 141, 143, 145, 146, 148, 152, 154, 157, 163, 168, 169, 171, 173, 177
neuropathic pain, 152
neuroprotection, ix, 128, 148, 157, 173, 175, 176, 181
neuroprotective agents, 144
neuroprotective drugs, 153
neuroscience, 153, 154, 162, 163, 167, 168, 173, 175, 176, 178, 180
neurotoxicity, 144, 147, 149, 154, 162, 164, 176, 179, 180
neurotransmitters, 179
nitric oxide, 129, 135, 137, 163
nitric oxide synthase, 129, 135, 137

nonsense mutation, 9, 21, 87, 92
non-small cell lung cancer (NSCLC), 93, 95, 96, 109, 110, 116, 117, 125
not otherwise specified (PTCL), 33, 76
Nrf2, 138, 144, 147, 163, 165, 169, 176
nucleic acid, 178
Nutlin, 22, 30, 31, 32, 39, 41, 53, 55, 56, 75, 125
nutrition, 177, 179

O

oligomerization, 3, 5, 6, 130, 131, 152, 159, 176, 178
oligomers, 2, 135, 146, 152, 178, 179
oncogene, viii, 35, 38, 42, 44, 57, 77, 83, 84, 101, 105, 108, 109, 116, 123, 124, 125, 167
ovarian cancer, 93, 96, 99, 100, 110, 117, 118, 121, 122, 124
oxidation, 129, 141
oxidative damage, 134, 138, 143
oxidative stress, v, viii, 2, 40, 74, 101, 127, 129, 136, 137, 154, 155, 156, 157, 158, 159, 160, 161, 162, 164, 165, 166, 167, 168, 169, 172, 173, 175, 179
oxide nanoparticles, 154
oxygen, 133, 144, 148, 150, 179, 180

P

p53 mutant, 15, 23, 32, 84, 88, 89, 97, 99
pancreatic cancer, 100
pathogenesis, viii, 9, 11, 21, 25, 36, 58, 65, 127, 135, 136, 152, 157, 174, 175
pathway, viii, 2, 3, 11, 13, 16, 19, 22, 23, 29, 30, 31, 33, 39, 40, 41, 48, 49, 57, 59, 69, 73, 74, 84, 86, 97, 100, 101, 140, 142, 143, 144, 146, 147, 151, 171, 173, 176, 180
peripheral blood, 32

peripheral T-cell lymphoma, 33, 54, 75, 76
permeability, 128, 133, 139, 176
pharmacology, 162, 169, 176, 179, 180
phenotype, 13, 33, 69, 88, 89, 93
pheochromocytoma, 141, 155, 160
phosphorylation, 3, 129, 131, 135, 137, 140, 144, 150, 151, 152, 154, 161, 165, 170, 175, 180
platelet derived growth factor receptor β (PDGFRβ), 100
polyubiquitination, 84, 102
prevalence, vii, viii, 2, 12, 15, 23, 28, 46, 83, 84, 93, 97
PRIMA-1^{MET} (APR-246), 19, 20, 23, 32, 40, 47, 58, 61, 69, 70, 99, 124
primary cells, 19
progenitor cell, 9, 13, 49
progenitor cells, 9, 13, 49
prognosis, viii, 7, 14, 30, 34, 36, 41, 43, 44, 50, 52, 57, 61, 65, 67, 72, 82, 83, 84, 89, 90, 91, 93, 95, 96, 101, 114, 115
pro-inflammatory, 144, 146, 149
proliferation, viii, 4, 9, 15, 31, 35, 36, 37, 73, 83, 86, 87, 89, 100
promoter, 3, 4, 5, 30, 38, 41, 130, 135, 167
proteasome, 18, 22, 38, 39, 41, 55, 68, 73, 84, 89, 99, 104, 111, 122, 148
protection, 138, 145, 160, 164, 180
protein kinase C, 144, 166
protein kinases, 128, 137
protein oxidation, 151
protein structure, 77
protein-protein interactions, 131
proteins, 13, 38, 41, 53, 65, 87, 131, 132, 134, 136, 138, 139, 146, 152, 154, 176

Q

quercetin, 141, 154, 155, 157, 158, 163, 164, 165, 170, 172, 181
query, 89, 90, 93

R

reactivation of p53 and induction of tumor cell apoptosis (RITA), 31, 39, 41, 56, 68, 69, 73, 79
reactive oxygen, viii, 127, 129, 132, 136, 180
receptor, 100, 133, 150, 151, 165
regeneration, 136, 156, 158, 160
relevance, 49, 64, 68
remission, 11, 17, 20
repair, 84, 100, 139, 179
repression, viii, 11, 64, 71, 127, 160, 165, 167
resistance, 7, 32, 40, 45, 56, 88, 96, 101
response, vii, viii, 1, 2, 3, 5, 7, 8, 14, 16, 17, 18, 20, 22, 24, 32, 37, 39, 46, 60, 84, 88, 91, 93, 96, 97, 99, 100, 127, 129, 131, 132, 133, 135, 138, 142, 150, 159, 167, 169
resveratrol, 148, 155, 160
risk, 7, 8, 10, 12, 14, 17, 20, 27, 36, 42, 53, 55, 59, 63, 66, 68, 76, 87, 92, 149

S

science, 75, 102, 103, 104, 105
senescence, 4, 37, 53, 61, 84, 108, 129, 150, 156, 181
sezary syndrome (SS), 34, 52, 78
signaling pathway, vii, viii, 2, 6, 30, 32, 39, 41, 84, 88, 141, 144, 150, 153, 159, 165, 179
SMZL, 25
solid tumors, vii, 1, 7, 22, 39, 51, 76, 89, 93, 94, 95
somatic mutations, 7, 14, 60
species, viii, 127, 129, 132, 136, 149, 167, 180
splenic marginal zone lymphoma (SMZL), 24, 25, 55, 64, 65
stress, 2, 3, 6, 8, 13, 33, 73, 84, 87, 133, 136, 151, 153, 155, 156, 160, 161, 167, 169
stress response, 136, 161
striatum, 145, 161, 177
structure, 5, 73, 141, 144, 152
subgroups, 13, 24, 43, 53, 54
superparamagnetic, 154
supplementation, 148, 162, 172, 180
suppression, viii, 4, 11, 13, 54, 88, 128, 161
survival, vii, 1, 3, 4, 8, 10, 12, 14, 23, 24, 28, 29, 30, 31, 32, 36, 37, 38, 42, 46, 47, 48, 51, 59, 62, 63, 67, 72, 73, 74, 76, 78, 81, 85, 86, 88, 89, 91, 92, 93, 95, 96, 97, 98, 131, 134, 138, 140, 141, 143, 146, 149, 166
syndrome, 7, 34, 49, 50, 51, 52, 57, 61, 67, 71, 78, 81, 152
synthetic lethality, 60, 98, 100

T

target, viii, 3, 4, 5, 6, 12, 13, 22, 30, 31, 37, 41, 46, 53, 75, 83, 84, 85, 87, 97, 98, 130, 134, 144, 146, 151, 152, 162, 166, 171
targeted therapy, 2, 16, 18, 19, 22, 30, 32, 38, 39, 40
targeting approaches, 98
tau, 135, 137, 141, 143, 145, 148, 150, 151, 152, 154, 159, 160, 161, 162, 165, 170, 171, 172, 173, 174, 175, 178, 180
The Cancer Genome Atlas (TCGA), 85, 86, 89, 90, 91, 94, 95
therapeutic agents, 41, 141
therapeutic approaches, viii, 2, 84
therapeutic effect, 19, 99
therapeutic strategies, 41, 98
therapeutic target, viii, 42, 46, 47, 74, 83, 84, 97, 98, 162
therapeutic targeting, 42, 47, 74, 84, 97, 98

Index

therapeutic targets, 162
therapeutics, 101, 153, 180
therapy, vii, 1, 2, 7, 8, 10, 15, 16, 18, 19, 20, 22, 23, 25, 30, 32, 33, 38, 39, 40, 46, 56, 64, 65, 75, 89, 92, 95, 97, 143, 153
therapy related AML (t-AML), 7, 8, 9, 12, 92
therapy related MDS (t-MDS), 7, 12, 92
toxic effect, 135
toxicity, 142, 145, 146, 147, 151, 153, 156, 165, 170, 180
TP53 deletion, viii, 1, 14, 21, 23, 25, 26, 27, 28, 29, 30, 32, 33, 34, 35, 36, 72
TP53 mutation, viii, 1, 5, 7, 8, 9, 10, 12, 13, 14, 15, 16, 20, 21, 23, 25, 26, 27, 28, 29, 30, 31, 32, 33, 34, 35, 36, 41, 42, 46, 47, 50, 53, 55, 57, 61, 63, 64, 66, 67, 69, 71, 72, 73, 84, 86, 87, 89, 91, 92, 93, 95, 96, 97, 102, 113, 114, 115, 116, 117, 118, 119, 120, 124
transcription, viii, 4, 5, 9, 56, 59, 68, 84, 87, 89, 127, 129, 130, 132, 133, 137, 138, 139, 144, 171, 178
transcription factors, 87, 89
transformation, 12, 14, 15, 16, 23, 25, 26, 31, 37, 44, 47, 50, 51, 64, 66, 68, 81
translocation, 21, 26, 27, 28, 132, 134, 139, 147
traumatic brain injury, 134, 161, 171
treatment, 13, 14, 15, 19, 22, 23, 24, 30, 31, 38, 39, 40, 45, 46, 53, 55, 56, 60, 61, 70, 96, 100, 101, 142, 143, 144, 148, 149, 152, 156, 167, 177
trial, 17, 18, 20, 22, 31, 39, 66, 76, 99, 100
tumor, viii, 2, 5, 9, 21, 26, 31, 32, 33, 35, 37, 39, 40, 44, 47, 57, 59, 62, 77, 83, 84, 85, 86, 87, 88, 89, 98, 129, 158, 166, 168, 169, 178, 179
tumor cells, 32, 40, 44
tumor growth, 32, 89
tumor progression, 129
tumor suppressor, viii, 2, 21, 26, 33, 35, 37, 44, 47, 57, 59, 62, 77, 83, 84, 85, 87, 89, 104, 111, 123, 158, 166, 168, 169, 178, 179
tyrosine, 22, 96, 100, 178

U

ubiquitin, 2, 3, 22, 38, 45, 84, 131, 139, 148, 150, 179
ubiquitinates, 84
ubiquitination, 2, 38, 39, 44, 99, 107
United States, 104, 106, 108, 109, 120, 121, 126, 168

V

variant allele of fraction (VAF), 10, 14, 15, 16, 91

W

wild type, 87, 88, 91, 92, 100

Z

zinc, 132, 136, 145, 150, 165, 180